Parenting
in the
Here and Now

Praise for *Parenting in the Here and Now*

How wonderful to open a book and feel that you have been invited into the author's home to experience the heart of her family life! Lea warmly and graciously engages her reader in her journey as a parent. With humour and candour, she encourages every parent not to try to be something that they are not, but rather to be the best that they already are. This book is an empowering guide to a truly heart-centered way of parenting.

Donna Simmons
Christopherus Homeschool Resources

Lea Page brings her warmth, her wit and her wisdom and walks with you heart-to-heart and side-by-side on the mysterious path of parenting. I wholeheartedly recommend this book to all grandparents, aunts, uncles, best friends, and teachers... everyone who loves a child and loves their parents.

Lynn Jericho
Mentor, Teacher, Writer (www.imagineself.com)

Lea Page points parents to a gentler path in her book *Parenting in the Here and Now*. She urges parents to face their fear and transform it to courage, a skill that allows presence of heart and mind for the most important job on the planet – ushering children into adulthood.

Lisa Groen Braner
Author of *The Mother's Book of Well-Being*

Parenting
in the
Here and Now

Realizing the Strengths
You Already Have

Lea Page

Floris Books

For Letter Man

First published in 2015 by Floris Books

© 2015 Lea Page
Lea Page has asserted her right under the
Copyright, Design and Patents Act 1988 to be
identified as the Author of this Work

 Also available
as an eBook

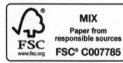

British Library CIP Data available
ISBN 978-178250-164-0

Printed in Great Britain
by Bell & Bain, Glasgow

Acknowledgements

To Tricia Mahlau-Heinert, Rachel Merrill, Jacquie Allman, Kimberly Rivera and Lisa Marshall, thank you for sharing the path and for the raucous, heartfelt and intelligent conversation. Thank you Jane Engebretzen, for your kindness. I am grateful to Melanie Lee for handing me my compass, ever so gently, and to Elizabeth Plant, for knocking on the door for me, one more time. Thanks to my father, Jake Page, who said, 'keep going,' and to my mother, Aida Bound, who listened when I kept on going and going. Thanks as well to Teresa Kiernan for her wholly biased editorial comments, to Dick Tinker, whose practical advice tamed the fearful "author bio" dragon, and to Ray and Rose Kuntz for their support. Elizabeth Stark Powers of Book Writing World welcomed me into her mentor group for new writers and opened up a whole world of possibility with her relentless positivity, and Judith Nasse, Thais Derich, Vijaya Nagarajan, Robert Ward, James Powers-Black, Devi Laskar, Bree LeMaire and Sylvia Foley inspired and humbled me with their courage and creativity. Thanks to Floris Books and especially to Eleanor Collins, my intrepid and good-humored editor.

To Nina and Thomas, my two greatest blessings, thank you for being so utterly yourselves and for teaching me so much about life and love. I am forever grateful for Ray, who makes me laugh every day. Thank you for having my back, for being at my side and, when necessary, for breaking trail during the storms. Words will never be enough.

Contents

**Part Three Parenting Challenges:
Ho Hum as a guide for discipline**

Conclusion

The beauty and the challenge of raising children is that even though all parents must make their way through virtually the same terrain, no two paths will ever be completely alike. With every child, the journey starts anew, its destination only revealed in glimpses for much of the way. Parents set out with hope, courage, love and a good helping of blind faith. *Parenting in the Here and Now* is a companion and guide for that journey. It shows the general lay of the land and what to watch out for: where the uphill climbs are, the roadblocks and the dead ends. For off-road travel – the bulk of the journey – there are principles for developing your own internal compass.

The path is yours to travel, but you need not do it alone.

Introduction:
What is Ho Hum?

This is Not a Fairy Tale

Once upon a time there was a mom, and every day she started over.

Every day she tried to live up to the image she had created for herself until one day she woke up and saw herself and her children without the haze of hope or wish or expectation or fear or disappointment, just saw them with clear eyes, with recognition, and because of that, the way was clear. There were no comparisons and no judgments, no 'shoulds' and no fear. She moved forward with clarity and confidence, and her children walked beside her. She realized that she had all she needed. Whatever might come her way, in her path, she had the eyes to see it, the language to speak to it and the strength to meet it.

The moral of the story: **You are already enough.** Remove a few obstacles and the path is clear.

You Are Already Enough

Are you going to be transformed by this book? I hope not. Here's why: this book is about how to use what you already have within you to be a more effective parent. It is not about remaking you into a different person.

Many of us parents wish to be transformed, some even believing that raising children is, in itself, a transformational experience. Certainly, we learn and grow ourselves as we nurture our children from infancy to adulthood. The desire to be transformed shows a willingness to sacrifice oneself, and it embodies the true depth of commitment parents have toward their children and the heights to which they will strive.

But the desire also harbors a hidden roadblock, which is the idea that you have to *be* some better version of who you are now. We are lured into thinking that we (and our children) are in a process of becoming better, that each step takes us onward toward a more perfect self. This idea leads to false conclusions. It implies that we somehow are not our true selves from the beginning.

Is the seed somehow less than the flower? It may have a different form, sure, but its essence is the same. It simply hasn't lived its whole life yet. Can we really say that the seed doesn't contain the flower? I don't think so. It is more that we can't see the flower yet. Every stage we go through is a necessary step in the unfolding of our selves. Be reassured that the parenting challenges you are facing right now are, simply, the fertile ground that will support that growth.

It is true that it can sometimes be worth trying new ways of *doing*. There are some changes that can make daily life with children run more smoothly and that might reduce your stress levels. We will talk about those things shortly, but they have nothing to do with changing who you *are*. That is most emphatically not the point. It is said that all we really have to offer at the end of the day – after dinner has been made, eaten and cleared away, after squabbles have been settled and laundry folded (or not!) – after all that, what we have left to offer is who we are. Yes, this is so. But why then would we substitute who we might be for who we are right now? Ought the seedling feel inadequate for not being in flower or fruit? Why strive towards being some imagined superior ideal?

Does this mean that you should never try to reach for the stars, never strive? No, not at all. It means that you can *do* all you want with who you are now. Rather than trying to perfect yourself by ignoring or denying some parts and accentuating others, aim to be more of who you are, not less. Instead of being selfless or selfish, be 'self-full.' Allow yourself the full measure of your being. This will enable you to harness capacities that you did not know you possessed, so that no matter what comes your way, you will be able to recognize it, understand it and deal with it as you must.

The Pythagoreans, the great thinkers of ancient Greece, did not carve 'Man, improve thyself' above the door to their place of study. Their words were: 'Man, know thyself; then thou shalt know the Universe and God.' The key to raising children is learning to see clearly and with imagination. It is uncovering and recognizing the whole self: our own whole selves and our children's. I don't mean that we are searching for a self that is whole. I mean that we are aiming to find the whole self: the sparks of uniqueness, the beauty and the strengths, and, as well, the flaws and the black holes that seem to always be hungry. For there is meaning to be found in all of it. Setting aside dreams of perfection in order to search out the true self unlocks the door to understanding, and, with that, parents can make better choices about how to proceed in any situation.

The bottom line is this: you can't fundamentally change who you are. People don't become better people. They learn to better use what they have. Mostly, this involves clearing away obstructions. So is there work to be done? Absolutely and always. But thinking that we must discard a part of ourselves or add something that we feel is missing is one of the greatest obstructions. Here, we are going to work on chipping away at that one, as well as a few others.

So this book does not seek to transform someone who has already been adequately supplied for her journey as a parent: that would be you. This book seeks to remove the obstacles that prevent you from clearly knowing yourself and your children. You will still have to walk the path yourself. It is your journey after all. Just remember: you are already enough.

Goals and Guilt

So, let's talk about guilt. Why now? Because guilt is paralyzing, and the last thing I want to do is present a perspective on parenting that leaves you feeling paralyzed. When I was a young mother reading parenting books and magazines, I would often be thrown into a paroxysm of guilt about yet another area in which I felt I had failed. Rather than considering how I might work with the new insight, I would endlessly kick myself around and around the block for what I hadn't known or understood. That was a big waste of time. But I was trying so hard to do right by my children, and my mistakes cut me to the core.

For the record: parenting involves making mistakes, sometimes *big* mistakes. Along with all of the laughs, stories and discoveries we share with our children, we also hit brick walls, say the wrong thing, do the wrong thing, and miss opportunities. I have done it. If you haven't yet, you surely will. We will talk more about mistakes later, but let me just say that mistakes are inevitable, and while we don't necessarily want to invite them over, we can work with them to our benefit when they do show up.

Guilt, on the other hand, has no business here. It shows up because we care so much. It infects us with subtle tentacles that insinuate themselves into our good intentions and undermine us with voices of doubt and second-guessing. Guilt makes us feel that it would be better if we just worked a little harder, were just a bit more this or had a bit more that. And that kernel of shame and of wishing that we were different than we are festers if we cover it over and allow it the darkness and silence in which it thrives.

The antidote is to bring in friends, especially the ones who have met that unwelcome party crasher themselves and recognize it for what it is, so that you and they can open it up to the light of day and flush it out with compassion and, sometimes, a good dose of humor. It requires vigilance, it requires courage and it requires persistence. We are all susceptible. Parents have such high expectations for themselves and their kids that frankly there is a lot of room for feeling like a failure, and sometimes rooting out the guilt can seem like an endless game of whack-a-mole. Our chief task is to love and to strive, always. Everything else is secondary. A positive mental outlook, athletic prowess, good hygiene habits, hand-knitted socks: all of those might be great things to give our children, but they are not on the list of absolute requirements.

My intention in writing this book is to offer you some thoughts and observations on raising children, along with a few all-purpose guiding principles that can be adapted to fit just about any situation. It is hard to do that, though, without implying that you could be a better parent, or worse, that you are not good enough right now... in other words, without opening wide the door to guilt. That is exactly what I don't want to do, and it is particularly difficult to avoid because I will be talking, at times, about some issues where I see a lot of misconception and misunderstanding.

Well, let's just say it: some things that we parents habitually do can lead to problems. I want to point out those things as well as suggest some alternatives, but understand that while you may be your own harshest critic (I certainly am mine), I am in no way in the business of judging you or anyone else. Judgment is simply irrelevant. We all struggle. We all have more to learn.

I want to tell you about a time when I was out for a hike with my son and a few other mothers and young children. I was still new to a small town in rural Montana, and this was one of the first times I had been invited to spend some time with these moms. I wanted things to go well. I wanted to make a good impression. I wanted to be liked; I wanted my son to be liked. Ah, yes. As you might imagine, it didn't turn out well.

We walked, we ate a picnic lunch in the woods, the children scurried about with their childish new eyes, the sun slanted through the trees and Rock Creek rushed and burbled. And my son, oh, he must have been about three, whacked one of the kids with a stick. I don't actually recall what happened immediately afterwards, what I did or said, but I remember the shoulder-slumping feeling, the deflation of hopes. He was in a rage about something and only got angrier as I attempted to diffuse the situation.

By this time, everyone was leaving. I remember, in the end, sitting down with him by the trail, holding him in my lap, encircling his flailing limbs with my own. He couldn't stop, and I could barely contain him. I almost had to sit on him to keep him from hurting me. And as I silently wrestled with him, praying for him to settle, each mother walked by me, silent as well, not even glancing at us. As the last mother passed by, though, she smiled the most cheerful, warm smile and said, 'It is hard to be a mom.' That's all.

That simple gesture, those few words, did so much for me. In that instant, I was not alone. I was not a disaster – or at least I was not the *only* disaster. She knew how hard it was, she knew how embarrassed I was, and she made it seem as if it was simply all in a day's work. No judgment. No worries. To say that she lifted my burden would be an understatement. By the time my son and I made it to the trail head where the rest were milling around the parking lot, instead of feeling like I wanted to hide in shame and never have to face any of those staring women again, I was able to make a joke about how I was a poor match in strength for a three-year-old boy.

We mothers need to do this for each other: see each other, recognize the work, the striving, the feelings and the loneliness in those moments of struggle. It matters. Averted eyes say more loudly than words ever could that whatever is happening would best be avoided. A word, a gesture, anything that says, 'I see you. I see you trying' – that is what we all need.

So that is what I am saying along with all the ideas and suggestions in this book. Simply: I see you trying. Yes, we all want help, we all want ideas, we all want a magic wand to solve everything, but before help and ideas can be effective we need to feel known and recognized.

Is This a Book for Mothers Only?

As you will see, I primarily address mothers. In writing this book, I imagined that you, the reader, and I are trusted friends who are out together, walking dogs and having a conversation. Over the course of my work and my life, I have had this conversation with countless people, most often with my own husband. I am speaking as I often do to mothers, but the conversation could just as easily and happily be with fathers, grandparents, teachers or anyone who has children in his or her life. I see you, too.

My Journey as a Parent

Many of those conversations happened along the dirt roads and mountain trails of rural Montana where my husband and I raised our children. My daughter was born in New York, and my first work with mothers began there through La Leche League, but we soon moved, stopping for a scant two years in New Mexico where my son was born,and landing in Montana.

Homeschooling afforded us the rare opportunity to spend the lion's share of our time together as a family. My husband, a country lawyer whose cases ranged from minors-in-possession to murder, taught our daughter and son math before driving to his office in town, where he was a sole practitioner. The children and I then spent the rest of the day immersed in our lessons: those of the book variety as well as those that are available when living in such wide-open beauty and grandeur.

With the Rocky Mountains and the Big Sky as our backdrop, we learned to differentiate the heron from the crane from a distance by the beat of their wings. We watched a mother moose, who gave birth to twins in our dry irrigation ditch, take her little ones out each day for a progressively longer walk until the day they left for good. My daughter rode her horse bareback over that same ditch, and my son built a giant bike jump over it (and only lost one layer of skin from his face while putting it to use). The choking wildfires of summer, the bounty from the garden in fall, the magical hoarfrost of winter and the return of the songbirds in the spring marked the passage of each year together.

For all the wonders of homeschooling, its greatest advantage was the gift of time. That was a period in our family life that I cherish. While there were many challenges for us in the outer world, the setting in which we lived was idyllic, and our life together on our twenty grassy acres was nearly so.

But it didn't start that way. Before even my first child was born, my goal was to be a good mother. It still is, but now I understand a little bit more about what that means. At that time, I had some pretty firm ideas about the kind of mother that I didn't want to be, and I was enthusiastic about the outcomes I imagined: my family would be harmonious and joyful and my children would be beloved and happy and creative and capable and... the list was pretty long. The fact that I was a bit fuzzy about how to get there seemed inconsequential at the time.

My husband and I assumed that our good intentions would see us through, and to some extent they did, but we ran into many of the problems that most well-meaning parents do. Despite a careful reading of the available books on parenting at the time, we kept on running into those same problems, over and over again. The obvious conclusion, I thought, was that there was something wrong with me. We would have muddled along as we were, and I would have continued to feel lost in the huge gap between the ideal that was presented in the books and the real me, had not something happened to change my perspective: my knight in shining armor (my husband) rode in to save the day, brandishing not a sword but a sense of humor.

Even the most challenging and rigid landscape will shift when you are laughing. My husband's jokes were the unvarnished truth, simple statements that revealed what would be obvious but for all of the accumulated assumptions obscuring it. When we spoke to our child as the books directed and our child did *not*, in fact, listen, my husband joked, '10,000 times is the charm,' and we laughed at the futility of it all. But when we were done laughing, I realized that we had overlooked the obvious: it *was* futile. No amount of talking would do the job. It was not a matter of finding the right *words* so that our child would listen; it was a matter of finding the right *action*. We had stumbled upon a truth about raising children, a reality that seemed patently obvious once we saw it.

When we peeled away that one assumption (that the right words were the answer to our parenting problems), other assumptions started to fall away as well. It seemed that once a little bit of light (or humor) was shone into the dark cave where our preconceived ideas and most of the conventional advice dwelled – unexamined and unchallenged – the problems that we were having, which we believed to be personal dragons, became ever so much more simple and manageable.

Another truth that we discovered standing right in front of us in broad daylight was that trying to superimpose calmness on top of anger and frustration made us more frustrated and angry! We had to learn what our emotions were really telling us. Then, instead of reacting out of emotion, we could harness their power to help us respond calmly.

A third truth emerged from these two: when we as parents stepped comfortably into our own authority, when we felt at home responding out of our understanding and experience, our capacity to take balanced action fell into place. Everyone was more at ease, and family life hummed along more harmoniously.

These truths form the basis of a parenting approach that we call 'Ho Hum.' It has a humble name because its principles are quite simple and humble themselves.

Ho Hum

Ho Hum is composed of three guiding principles. The first involves understanding the role your emotions play so that you aren't overwhelmed by fear, anger and guilt. This understanding can help you respond calmly in stressful situations. Calmness opens the gateway to strengths you might not know you have, strengths that form the foundation of parental authority: your caring and understanding, and your wisdom and experience. Realizing these capacities helps you to be comfortable in your parental authority, which is the second principle of Ho Hum. And finally, the third principle involves communicating with the language of authority. It is a language that allows you to avoid power struggles and which children understand naturally: it is a language of actions and experiences rather than words.

The overarching purpose of Ho Hum is to enable you to act instead of react.

The three principles, as you will have gathered from my descriptions of them, are connected – each reinforces the others. Using actions rather than words will assist you in keeping calm and will help you step into parental authority. Understanding your emotions and responding calmly gives mental space for acting and enables a more balanced parental authority. Being comfortable with your authority leads to calmer responses and a focus on what happens next rather than endless debate.

I believe that Ho Hum is at the heart of raising children: no matter what your specific approach is, Ho Hum is your compass. No matter where your journey as a parent takes you, Ho Hum will help you find your way.

How This Book is Organized

Parenting in the Here and Now has three main parts.

Part One addresses the principles of Ho Hum, the foundation for harmonious family life. The first chapter explores our parental anger, guilt and fear, and shows how we can acknowledge those emotions so they don't obstruct our vision and our actions. The second chapter describes healthy parental authority, without which we cannot act effectively. The nature of words and the pitfalls of relying on them when caring for children are exposed in Chapter Three. A vital example of Ho Hum in action is shown in Chapter Four, where I suggest we make choices for our young children rather than offer choices to them.

Part Two addresses the environment in which our daily parenting takes place. It discusses ways of setting up a household and a family life that are conducive, in my experience, to helping things run more smoothly. In Part Two, Chapter Five is about rhythm – having a pattern in daily life so that there is some predictability and much of what needs to happen has a flow, requiring no negotiation. Chapter Six covers chores and our expectations of children's participation in the running of the household. Chapter Seven focuses on how we can think about play so that it is likely to work well for children and parents. These chapters challenge common assumptions about what children need. Those assumptions are responsible for many obstacles, but with a bit of awareness you can set them aside and proceed with more freedom and ease.

Part Two has ideas about how to set up family life, space and expectations so that conflicts and challenges are rarer, but no matter how strong your foundation, things inevitably will go wrong at times. Part Three contains many practical examples for using the approach of Ho Hum when you are faced with particular parenting problems, from tantrums to lies, from disrespect to resistance. Part Three gives many examples for how to shift from talking at our kids, to actions and experiences that allow them to genuinely learn from their mistakes and misbehavior. While no one book can address every issue or problem that parents will face, the principles of Ho Hum can be applied broadly to any difficulty, and the many examples through Part Three will help you grasp how to do this.

The book's conclusion offers some suggestions about how to take the first steps if you would like to bring the Ho Hum approach into your own family life. It poses questions that you can ask yourself, so that you can find your own answers.

One more thing. Consider any thoughts here with this question in mind: do they feel right and make sense to you? You get to decide what will work for you. These perspectives are *my* truths, but I would never claim that they are absolute truths. I am offering them here for you to sample, taste, wolf down or spit out. Since I believe that we all are striving in our own way, I would like to present what follows in the spirit of an ongoing conversation, one that you may have been having with yourself and perhaps with others and will continue to have. There is great joy and wonder to be had in raising children, but it is not an easy path. So let's walk it together here, for a little while, and see if I can shine a bit of light so that is it easier for you to find your way. No judgment. No worries.

Part One

Ho Hum – The Three Principles

Chapter One
Being Calm

Ho Hum is a way to approach difficulties. It is the acceptance of the tasks at hand, the addressing of concerns in a matter-of-fact way, the attendance to the needs of the moment without getting caught up in emotional storms. It is responding in a measured, considered way. For parents, it is the closest thing we will ever have to a magic wand. The principles of Ho Hum are:

1. Be calm;
2. Be confident in your parental authority;
3. Respond with actions and experiences rather than words.

It is an approach which, as a young parent, I desperately needed.

An example: I am seated beside my young daughter, her legs tucked neatly while mine are bent at odd angles to fit around the child-sized table. With sheets of colored paper stacked at our elbows, we lean our chins on our cupped hands as we study the cryptic directions: Fold corner A to corner B. Crease. Open; rotate; repeat. It sounds easy enough at the beginning. She selects royal blue. I take canary yellow. Our objective: an origami bird. My dad used to make them all the time. There are easier shapes to start with, but Nina has her heart set on the bird: it has so much more grace than the cup or the frog. What is the worst that could happen?

I slide over a third sheet and fold it in half, lining up the corners and edges with exaggerated care before pressing down the crease. 'It is tricky,' I say. 'Let's practice a bit before we get started on the real thing.'

PART ONE: THE THREE PRINCIPLES OF HO HUM

Nina will have none of that, so I shrug, and we begin. I read out the directions for the first step. We both fold and crease. So far, so good. I read out the next steps, and we continue folding. I remind her about the need for care in lining up the edges.

'I know, Mom,' she says, as she slides her pudgy little thumb across a crumpled crease. Her corners are decidedly askew, but I don't want to harp on her too much. It doesn't need to be perfect. As we progress, her paper resembles the neat drawings less and less. 'It's all messed up,' she says, chin quivering, useless hands hanging down at her sides.

'Here, let's see,' I offer, as I set my half-done bird down and reach for hers. And so we slip over the edge and hurtle down the slope towards disaster. I hear my voice becoming more plaintive as each suggestion I make is dismissed. She is simultaneously defeated and defiant, and I am at the end of my rope. She sobs and, feeling helpless, I open my hands out in frustrated supplication and say, 'Why won't you just let me help you?'

'Because nothing you do ever helps,' she wails.

I suck in my breath, the gulp of air fanning into flames the embers of my inadequacy. I clench my teeth. My eyes narrow and bore into hers. I count off on my fingers all the different ways that I tried to help her fix or redo her bird, and I growl, 'And you think that wasn't being helpful?' And in a flight of sheer bug-eyed rage, I say, 'I will show you what isn't helpful,' and I snatch her misshapen wad of paper, and with a dramatic flourish, I crush it in my hand.

For a moment, we are both paralyzed, shocked. Did I really just do that? She breaks the silence by crumpling into a devastated heap, and I am horrified at myself. There is no more rage, just regret, and I hold her and rock her and apologize over and over. It is a long time before she settles down, but she won't look at me for even longer. What have I done? How could I have gotten so angry over origami?

Had I understood it then, Ho Hum could have been the lifeboat I so sorely needed at that embarrassingly low moment. My daughter and I might not have gotten any further with our paper folding, but Ho Hum would have enabled me to surface and gain a breath of perspective, which in turn would have kept me off the emotional roller coaster that I rode to such a spectacularly disastrous finish.

This chapter is about the first principle of Ho Hum, which is: be calm.

'Oh, sure,' you might be thinking, 'it's easy enough to *say* "be calm." As a recommendation, it's obvious to anyone. None of us ever *plan* on losing our cool and yelling at our kids.'

You are right to be skeptical. When advice is easy to give but hard to follow, it just sets us up for failure. I certainly was trying to remain calm about the origami, and to say that I failed would be a profound understatement. There had been times when I was able to maintain my self-control when I was upset, but despite my valiant and persistent efforts, there continued to be many failures, although, thankfully, none were quite as dramatic as the one above. It seemed that I could only get so far, hold on for so long, before something would blow. What I later discovered was that there is a world of difference between adopting the Ho Hum approach to being calm and managing to hold back a storm through sheer force of will.

Having self-control seems like a worthy goal, but it actually misses the whole point. It doesn't work for you to be calm on the outside if you aren't calm on the inside. With Ho Hum, you respond in a calm manner because you *are* calm, not because you are able to *appear* calm despite being in turmoil.

So now, it seems, the bar has been raised even higher: it is no longer good enough to just keep your cool when you are at the end of your rope. Somehow, you must not even get upset, as if you have an endless supply of rope so that you never reach the end of it. If you can't manage the first goal, how could you possibly manage the second?

It seems so unrealistic, but let's look more closely at these emotions we are trying so hard to control.

Our Emotions Have a Role – Even Anger

Some of us yell. Some of us snap. Some of us cry. Some of us combine all of these and more when we lose our self-control. It all stems from being overloaded by emotion, and the emotion most commonly present at the flash point is anger. Does this mean that we have to deny our emotion, hide it or shut ourselves off from it? Absolutely not. Emotion, and anger in particular, plays a crucial role. Emotion is the first manifestation, our first reading, of all of the sensory information that we absorb both consciously and sub-consciously. Like a reflex, it is much quicker than our thoughts, which is why we so often have a gut feeling about something or someone before we really understand why. Without our emotion, we would be lost.

Emotion in general is a signal that draws our attention. More than any other emotion, anger in particular serves us by being a red flag, warning us that all is not well. Since it is one of our most reliable indicators that trouble is afoot, we ignore it at our peril, but, paradoxically, anger also gives us extremely unreliable information about where to go to find solutions. It doesn't even steer us in the direction of the real problem, often pointing us toward the nearest, easiest target for expediency's sake. Anger (and its pal, resentment) need to be taken seriously, but we don't necessarily want to follow where they indicate.

Anger itself is not a problem; the problem comes when we ignore its first warning flash. For parents, this can happen because we are tired or busy, but it frequently happens because we are too patient. 'What?' you might say. 'I have been trying to be *more* patient and *less* angry!' This is backwards, and that is why it never works. We have all been taught that patience is a virtue, and in many contexts it is, but all things have a light and a dark side, and the dark side of patience is thinking that one must ignore one's sense of wrongness. We mistakenly believe that patience means putting up with or learning to live with a problem. As we all know, when we do that, anger, our devoted early warning system, does not shrink quietly away. If it is not noticed and addressed, anger will re-assert itself, usually at a time when we are more vulnerable and less able to stuff it away, and that is when we blow up. Because we have waited until we are at the end of our rope, we cannot separate our feelings about its message from our action based on the message.

If we take proper note of our emotions as signals and give them the respect that they deserve, we will not be at their mercy. Combined with our ability to step back and analyze, our emotions are an essential part of our decision-making process. Responding to difficulties with Ho Hum depends on our ability to understand the role that emotion rightly plays.

Anger is part of a sprawling family and has many cousins: desperation, guilt, exhaustion, loneliness, helplessness, inadequacy. We could call them a sorry cast of characters, but remember: they are all messengers, not permanent guests. If we listen respectfully and attentively to what they have to say, they will leave of their own accord. So let's invite them all in for a moment and have a good look. When we take the opportunity to observe them calmly from across the kitchen table, as it were, instead of over our shoulders with the whites of our eyes showing, we may notice that they share a strong family resemblance. Yes, anger blusters and guilt shrinks, but they are all, in the end, offspring of one common ancestor, one who rarely makes its presence known but sends the others as proxies. And who might that be? Let me introduce you to fear, although you have probably already met.

At the Root of It: Fear

Fear sends us careening down the path that dead-ends with yelling and tears. Feeling frustrated, tired and stuck? We can usually handle our share of this and more. It is the addition of fear, and its handmaiden guilt, that turns difficult-but-manageable into impossible.

We may feel tired and frazzled after a long day when we are stuck in traffic and are late to pick up our child at daycare and have to stop at the grocery store on the way home. When she has a meltdown in the checkout line, not only are we embarrassed, but we feel guilty that she too is having an overly long and stressful day, and beneath that, we fear that this will somehow do her harm, and so we bark at her and pull her roughly from the cart. We may be frustrated when our child clings to us and refuses to look at, let alone play with other children, but it is fear that she will never feel comfortable in social situations that pushes us to snap. As she sits at the table, struggling with a math problem, our inability to explain may make us feel impatient, but it is our fear that she will never get it and will therefore have limited opportunities that leads us to our feeling of inadequacy and our disparaging comments. We may feel helpless when she needs more and still more from us at a time when we ourselves are emotionally depleted, but the roar of anger that gives us some much-needed space comes on the heels of fear, which whispers to us that we will never be that better person who always has a bit left in reserve.

Let's look closer at that long day filled with traffic and errands when we are tired and frazzled. Without feeling guilty that things are disjointed, and without feeling fearful that it will affect our child badly, we could accept that it is, no more and no less, a bad day. It isn't what we would have wanted, but here it is. Ho Hum. We could allow ourselves to be tired. We could make a less-than-perfect dinner. We could leave the laundry in the basket unfolded. Without the fear goading us, we can recognize – and more importantly, *accept* – what we can and can't do that day. It is, after all, only reality.

With Ho Hum, we concern ourselves with what is literally before us at the moment. Sometimes that includes being tired and frazzled. Guilt and fear tell us that nothing short of the ideal will suffice. The more we can **attend to the 'what is' of the moment and not the 'what I wish it were' or the 'what it should be,'** the easier it will be to step back and assess what we might possibly do differently next time.

Ironically, allowing yourself to simply attend to the moment at hand gives you a doorway out of it. Your feelings of being angry, resentful, stressed and overwhelmed by your day are the emotional messengers telling you that some adjustments might need to be made. Fear and guilt insinuate that the adjustment must be in who you *are*, which gives rise to more fear and guilt – a reasonable reaction since there really is very little you can do to change your very being. Ho Hum, on the other hand, guides you to adjust what you *do*. It is harder than you might think to change what you do, but it is possible, and it is ultimately the *only* thing that is possible.

Clearly, the key to being calm and not just appearing so, is connected to fear. But we can't just not be fearful.

Consider this: think about the last time your child had the stomach flu (and if you have yet to experience this, I don't want to gross you out, but you might as well be prepared, since it will happen eventually).

Your child is at the dinner table, grumpy, pale and listless. At the end of the meal, during which she hardly eats, she refuses to clear her plate, and before you can open your mouth to remind her, she opens hers and vomits in her lap. Do you get mad or upset? No. This is the time for action, and the sooner the better. You set aside the dishes you were carrying, grab her and rush to the bathroom where you hold her hair back from her face and put a hand gently on the small of her back.

Shocked you may be, disgusted too at the mess waiting for you in the kitchen, but right now you murmur, 'There, there, it will be all right.' When she is done, you help her out of her soiled clothes, grab a towel to place over her pillow, put her in her pjs and tuck her into bed, racing out and coming back with a bucket. There is the mess of her clothes on the bathroom floor, the bigger mess at the table, and you don't even want to think about what the dog is doing, but right now you sit on the edge of her bed, soothing her as she hiccups and whimpers.

Eventually, she drifts off to sleep, and, knowing that it is not over yet, you dash out, leaving her door open so you can hear her when she wakes. You head to the bathroom, but before you have brought all the clothes and dirty towels to the washing machine, your daughter cries out and retches again. You drop the laundry basket and rush back to her room, holding the bucket for her, reassuring her that as awful as it is right now, it will pass. As you wait for this bout to run its course, you think about all the things that you need to do to be prepared for a long night with little sleep.

This will be a test of endurance. You may feel sorry for your child, sorry for yourself, even. You may feel frustrated that whatever you had planned to do that night will have to be put off until another time. Plans for the next day will have to be cancelled. But there is nothing for it. The circumstances demand an adjustment, and you make it. Ho Hum.

It bears repeating: **circumstances demand an adjustment and you make that adjustment.** You are acting out of necessity, not reacting out of emotion. The emotions are surely there, but in this situation, they tend to take a back seat because the imperative of action is so strong. No matter what, you will have to let this one run its course. The most you can hope for is to stay on top of the laundry, and even that may be a stretch. Comforting and caring for your child comes first. You may be resigned. You may even be exhausted and a little short-tempered, but there is no judgment and no blame. The circumstances are beyond your control, so you simply respond as the circumstances require and as you are able.

You respond to an illness like this as you would any force of nature. You may be feeling all manner of emotions, *and* you do what you need to do. That is Ho Hum.

The Role of Fear

Our fear exists because our children are so important to us. We love them beyond description, and when things go wrong, we fear that we are not up to the task of helping them, protecting them, or guiding them. We fear that our past mistakes have caused harm, which leaves us feeling guilty, and we fear that if we do the wrong thing now, their future may be irreparably damaged. When our sweet children appear selfish, lazy, dishonest or rude, we worry: what if they never learn? What if they never overcome their faults and weaknesses? What if they continue to make the same mistakes or worse? Such pressure we put on ourselves. It is a wonder that on some days, we don't curl up in a ball and hide.

Yes, we have a desire to do what is right, what is best. We have a responsibility as well, a duty even, yet out of the love that inspires us and motivates us also comes fear. Fear is our greatest obstacle, but only because we don't understand it. Like anger, we can learn to recognize it and, more importantly, distinguish what it means from what it says. Most often, **fear says: 'You are guilty. You have failed. You are no good. You are not enough.'** What fear *means* is: 'This matters. Your child matters. You matter.'

When we only hear what fear *says* ('...wrong, inadequate, inferior...'), we may be paralyzed, or we may react out of the cascade of emotions that we very legitimately feel, and in either case we often respond in ways that we later regret. The true message that fear brings is lost on us. When we understand what fear *means* ('You are the one. This is the time. Have courage.'), something entirely different happens. We do not become paralyzed or lost to our emotions. We *focus.*

We see with clarity what is before us. We set aside the extraneous, the less important, the things that can wait. Our hand is steadied. Whether we are absolutely sure or not, we act because we know that we must. If we make mistakes, we make them with confidence, knowing that we must do the best we can with what we know and see and have available to us in this moment. We know that later, if we have more information or understanding or just plain hindsight, we can adjust our course, again doing the best we can with what we have at that next moment. This is all we can ever do. This is Ho Hum.

Whether we are whisking our eighteen-month-old child upside

down and pounding her back to dislodge the piece of apple that is choking her, or are listening to our eighteen-year-old college student weeping over the phone, we are focused on this moment and this moment only. The guilt about yesterday or last year? That is extraneous right now. Worrying about our child's table manners, or whether our teen will ever settle on a career path when she can't settle on a class schedule, can wait.

This is Ho Hum. This **focus on the needs of this moment and only this moment** is what enables us to listen, to respond, to do what needs to be done, no matter how scary or difficult it is, and to be calm while we do it. We are clear. In a paradoxical way, we are removed a step from the situation, enough so that we can observe it, including our emotions, with greater perspective, but at the same time, **we are more present than ever because we are not distracted by our emotions. We have heard their warning, and now we can thank them with grace and set them aside to be attended to again later when we are not so pressed. We only need carry the weight of now.** And with our arms less encumbered, we have so much more strength to bring with us to the task at hand. Instead of squandering our energy by resisting and denying our emotions, we can hear them gratefully and then let them go, so that our hearts can be filled with love as we turn to face whatever challenge is before us.

Fear, which we thought was our great enemy, can be an ally. If we are attentive to it rather than driven by it and we hear its message to focus, to focus on the here and now, that can help bring us to being calm, the first principle of Ho Hum.

What Ho Hum has to Offer

Approaching difficulties with Ho Hum doesn't guarantee that you will always be successful. There are no guarantees. What it does do is enable you to do the best that you can in any given moment. Informed by your emotions but not driven by them, you understand and accept the realities of what you have before you: a screaming baby, a dejected child, a sullen teenager, an ill spouse, a tired self. You consider your options, make a decision, and then you proceed as best you can. Ho Hum.

Like a force of nature, raising children brings with it inevitable patterns of joy and success, challenge and failure. We can count on that, just as we expect the sun to rise in the morning and set in the evening. Challenges, problems and crises will come, not because of who we are or who we are not, but because that is just part of raising children. The road, when we can find it, is not always smooth. Ho Hum is a helpful companion and sometimes is a lifesaver.

So let's go back to the origami incident and see how it might have turned out differently if I had had a good helping of Ho Hum. Keep in mind that I am not judging myself through the lens of my hindsight. That is never fair, nor is it realistic: I didn't know then what I know now (and knowing my daughter better now, I would never have embarked on such a project to begin with when it was almost certainly beyond her abilities). But going through the exercise of revisiting my mistakes, of seeing where I got off-track, is definitely worthwhile. It may help me to recognize sooner the next time I start to lose my way.

Again, we are seated at our little table with our sheets of colored paper. Fold corner A to corner B. Crease. It sounds easy enough. What is the worst that could happen? 'It is tricky,' I say. 'Let's practice a bit before we get started on the real thing.' Nina will have none of that, so I shrug. I notice little pricks of anxiety: 'Is this going to work?' We begin. Her corners are decidedly askew, but I don't want to harp on her too much. It doesn't need to be perfect. As we progress, her paper resembles the neat drawings less and less.

'It's all messed up,' she says. The feeling of anxiety turns to guilt: I should have known that this wouldn't work. Am I a failure? It is tempting to think so, to sink into self-pity, to make this project a referendum on my worth. I feel anger rising: if Nina would just let me fix it, we could snatch success from defeat, I will no longer be a failure and I can reassure myself that I am a good mother.

But this time I pause as the emotions cascade over me. The guilt, the disappointment, the anger are pounding at the door. Ho Hum, I think to myself. I knew this might not turn out well, and still I am feeling so badly. What is really going on here? And I say it to myself: 'I feel like a complete failure.' I open the door, letting it all in, and allow myself a moment to just howl inwardly in frustration. I am shocked at myself, but there it is. My guilt is simmering still. I can feel it in my stomach, and I want desperately to purge myself of it somehow.

But I am also aware of reality: somehow, watching that parade of emotion marching past me allows me to look past it to what actually is before me now. It is simple, really. We have bitten off more than we can chew. I have made a mistake in choosing a project that does, in fact, require a certain amount of precision, if not perfection. I clearly have a lot – too much – invested in this. I am feeling rotten, *and* I need to attend to what is happening right now. Despite my emotion's insistence that it is all about me, the truth is, Nina is the one in trouble. She is a little girl who is stuck, and while it truly feels like the world has come to an end, it is *just paper.* Do I want her to feel that the outcome is the most important thing? It only has to be a big deal if I make it so.

I look at my daughter sitting there, tears threatening, and I slap my hand to my forehead and state the obvious, 'This is *so* hard. I knew it would be tricky, but I had *no* idea.' I can feel the weight lifting from me. We can fail. No big deal. Ho Hum. 'Here, let's see,' I offer, as I set my half-done bird down and reach for hers.

It turns out that Ho Hum doesn't give me magic origami powers. I am still unable to help my daughter salvage her crane, and she is still not particularly appreciative of my efforts, even though this time they are offered without the extra dose of my frustration and without my self-worth hanging in the balance. In fact, she still wails that nothing I do ever helps. Ho Hum. I am not a failure; I am needed. Her emotional reaction tells me so. There is work to do here, and in doing it, I am redeemed.

She is really upset. I see that there *is* nothing I can do to help with the paper. I pull her into my lap and circle my arms around her, and she cries. I am not tight with emotion. I have let it go. Maybe we can try again later, maybe not. It is what it is: a poor choice of activities that didn't turn out as expected. No more, no less.

I had envisioned sharing a pleasant moment together with my daughter, where we would both be swept along on a current of colored paper and beautiful, graceful creations. Our reality doesn't quite match that ideal. The circumstances require an adjustment. The more I cling to my ideal, the more the gap between it and our reality becomes a black hole of judgment: a sink that can never be filled. Ho

Hum simply points out to me in a rather matter-of-fact way that while the ideal was nice, I am dealing with something else today. If I have made a poor choice with the origami, then we will have to do the best we can at muddling through. It was a mistake, not a moral failing.

My fears whispered to me that I would never be able to help her in the way that she needed, that my mistakes and failings would cause her harm. Ho Hum points out that while that may or may not be true, in this moment, this very moment, I can help her best by not getting caught in those worries. I can help her best by letting go of the wish for 'how it might be' and by responding to 'how it is.' By approaching my failure with Ho Hum, I am showing her how to approach her failure with Ho Hum, and no folded crane is more valuable than that.

This is Ho Hum: acceptance of and adjustment to 'what is.' Our emotional reaction is part of what is. When we learn its language, we understand that it is urging us to focus and to act.

What Ho Hum is Not

Let me clarify: Ho Hum is about accepting the tasks at hand, but this acceptance might be misconstrued to mean accepting a problem, i.e., allowing it to continue. Or accepting one's anger or disappointment, meaning learning to live with it. This is the antithesis of Ho Hum.

Think of the acceptance in Ho Hum as the willing acceptance of a challenge or of an invitation to an event in which you are the main actor. Acceptance means that you agree to be present. Ho Hum does *not* mean pretending that the trail of cast-off shoes, jackets and overflowing backpacks between the front door and the kitchen isn't making you grind your teeth when you come home with arms full of grocery bags. Ho Hum means that you take note of your irritation and resentment, you step back a moment (or several moments if need be) to consider what the problem is and where the heart of it lies, and then you act with love, warmth and firmness, and perhaps, on the best of days, with a little humor and grace, although we can't always expect miracles. Ho Hum is not about swallowing, absorbing, reacting or rejecting. It is about acting; it is about moving forward.

Ho Hum is also not a new ideal with which to bludgeon yourself if you cannot always attain it. The concept itself is difficult to grasp. Learning how to put it into practice takes a lifetime. It is a huge challenge and a hugely rewarding one, but it won't come easily. You must start small. Give it a try sometime with something relatively inconsequential, where you can get a little feel for it. Or, as life would have it, you may find yourself in a right mess and figure that now is as good a time as ever to jump in and give it a go.

Know this: it takes practice. Lots of practice. You will need to be very patient with and forgiving of yourself. Be observant and a little curious. Notice where you slip and why. Give a shrug and accept your failures and half-starts as part of the learning process. Take heart and have courage to wade back in and try again. Accept this challenge with as much love and good grace as you can muster. The difficulties will present themselves, that we know. (As my husband says, 'The fun never stops!') You can meet those difficulties the hard way or the Ho Hum way.

Ho Hum is not an easy way, but I assure you that it does get easier. You will have lots of opportunities to develop it. And just so you know, in the time that it took me to write this chapter, I had several chances to put Ho Hum to use. The seemingly more difficult one involved my daughter, who was in Cameroon and who became quite ill and was taken to the hospital. Despite having no internet, and phone service that was spotty at best, I was able to navigate that one.

On the other hand, I had a total breakdown about the fact that we still haven't been able to replace a disgusting and malfunctioning toilet after seven months. Go figure. I know what was simmering beneath that one and will have an opportunity to try again. Sometimes the best we can do is to achieve Ho Hum retrospectively, acknowledging our mistakes and making a plan so that the next time we will do better (remember: *do* better, not *be* better).

Let me be clear: **working towards Ho Hum is a life's work. It takes attention, constant attention, and a willingness to wade back in when you have drifted away and are having your own version of an 'origami' moment. Learning to listen to fear, anger and guilt, learning to understand what they mean rather than what they immediately say, and learning to act, not in spite of their presence but in addition to their presence, takes practice – a lifetime of practice.** Ho Hum is a *real* fix, but it is not a *quick* fix.

Where to Start

When you are feeling overwhelmed, you can help yourself focus on the immediate moment by asking: **What does my child need from me right now?**

Greet your emotions as they arrive, 'Oh, hello Frustration. You are here because this is the gazillionth time I have had to pull these two squabbling children apart, and frankly, I have had it. Hello, feelings of Failure and Guilt, you are here because, if I were to admit it, I blame myself for my kids' continual fights. But if you will excuse me for a moment, I have a job to do.'

When faced with a difficulty, ask, 'What am I fearing? What is the worst that I can imagine?' You might as well get to the heart of it. Don't dismiss the fear – it always has merit – but draw it alongside, so you can be on a first name basis with it.

Often, you will have to do this retrospectively, when you are thinking about something that already happened: 'What was I fearing?' Keep practicing this step. Look at the fear. The more you notice it and the longer you can look at it with a steady gaze, the less you will feel driven by it and the more you will find you are calm. Not trying to appear calm, but being calm.

If you have regularly occurring events that set you off, plan for them in advance by imagining how you will feel. Notice who shows up: do you expect Loneliness, Inadequacy and Fear? Be aware of them now. Listen to what they say, and then remember what they mean: 'This is important. *Focus.*'

AND THEN, do the best that you can do with what you know and have at that moment. That is all any of us can ever do, and that is enough.

Chapter Two
Being Confident in Your Parental Authority

Once again the principles of Ho Hum are:

1. Be calm;
2. Be confident in your parental authority;
3. Respond with actions and experiences rather than words.

This chapter is about the second of these principles. It discusses finding a degree of parental authority that works for you, being able to adapt it to circumstances and, most importantly, being able to step into it confidently. It is about knowing with certainty that in any situation that arises, *you* are the parent, *you* are the one with life experience and a relationship to this child, *you* are the one with the authority to act.

Between Calm and Action

So here we are, with our anger and our fear right there beside us, invited in, so to speak. They don't have to sneak in through the back door, worrying us by making a din in the kitchen while we are trying to put up a good front in the living room. Our reluctance to invite them to the party, to bring them forward into the light of day, gave them power, and it took so much energy to hold them off, to resist. But somehow, once we have looked them squarely in the eye, we understand that they are not actually here to hinder us but to bolster us, to stand with us as we turn towards the matter at hand, whatever it is.

With fear beside us, reminding us to focus on what is right before us, and *only* that, we find that we do, indeed, have a deep reservoir of calmness. Instead of being driven by anger, crushed by guilt or paralyzed with fear, instead of coming apart at the seams, we feel solid and grounded. Our feet feel firmly planted on the ground, and from that, we can draw strength.

Is this a bit of overkill for, say, responding when your child has left his dirty dishes around for the umpteenth time or refuses to put his jacket on and get in the car? Maybe on a good day you won't need the sense of strength and serenity that comes with knowing that fear is not sneaking up behind your back but is actually watching it for you. But on a bad day? You may find that having Ho Hum is the difference between a bad day and a nightmare. Sometimes it is the most seemingly inconsequential bumps in the road that have the potential to bring us to our knees: a half-done origami bird, perhaps, or a backed-up toilet. We stumble, and in doing so, we lose our bearings and forget what we know. No moment is too insignificant for Ho Hum.

Now that we are calm, we must turn our attention to the needs of this moment: our children who are bickering or not doing their homework, who are unable to ride a bike or make friends, who come home too late at night or smelling of alcohol. We must act. With a deep breath for courage, we put our hands on our hips, and face forward, prepared for whatever it is that lies in our path.

But there are so many pathways. There is a whole spectrum of parenting approaches, all with their vocal proponents. How are we to choose?

The Spectrum of Parenting Approaches

At one end of the spectrum is the so-called 'tiger' mom. She sets extraordinarily high standards in all areas for her children and then proceeds to drive them relentlessly to meet those standards. She is convinced that through the force of her will, she can shape her children to meet her expectations. Seeking to control the future, she leaves nothing to chance. Her children will have no flaws and no weaknesses. It simply will not be permitted. She will tolerate nothing short of perfection and complete obedience, and her children often reward her efforts with exceedingly high achievements in the areas which she has chosen.

She believes she is helping her children to succeed in a harsh and competitive world where the spoils go to the few who can reach the top. In order to protect her children from the pain of failure, she herself will cross the line into abuse. By seeing her children as empty cups to be filled – by her – she never knows who her children are. Their beings exist only as a kind of slave to or reflection of her will.

On the other side of the spectrum is the 'free market' mom. This parent does not impose her expectations on her children. Exerting no will in order to influence them, she takes no responsibility for guiding their behavior or their future. She believes that flaws and weaknesses are caused by parents meddling unduly with their children's innate wisdom. She thinks that any exertion of parental will corrupts children's free will, which, she also believes, if left on its own, will flourish and become self-correcting. Ironically, this approach produces children whose cups are so full of their own being that there is little room for anything else, and they become the tyrants she has tried so hard to avoid being herself.

The 'tiger' mom will not allow any flaws or mistakes in her children; the 'free market' mom will not recognize any flaws or mistakes in her children. Both types of parent must deny a considerable amount of reality in order to adhere to their preferred approach. As with fundamentalism in politics or religion, there is a high price to pay in reaching for their narrow, utopian ideals.

These parents' convictions are usually confirmed when they try a taste of the opposite end of the spectrum. The 'tiger' mom, momentarily bowing to popular pressure to 'let her kids be kids,' allows a freedom where she never had before. The result, all too often, is that her children are simply at a loss. Having always been told what to do, when they are given a moment of freedom, they don't know what to use it for, and may, sadly, respond with dismay. The 'tiger' mom observes their paralysis and sees it as further evidence that her children need her to direct their every moment.

The 'free market' mom, probably tired of picking up after her 'free' children, decides to implement a bit of expectation. She informs her children that they will, in fact, be responsible for something, and they, predictably, refuse. She has, after all, taught them that they are their own highest authority. Against such resistance, it would take relatively draconian measures (she believes) to get them to meet even the most modest expectation. The ensuing misery confirms her belief that parental expectations lead to problems.

Most parents find themselves somewhere between these two far ends of the spectrum. Well, the reality is that many parents find themselves swinging back and forth between them. It is hard to find the right balance. You know how it is: we have an image of how things might be, and so we set ourselves, if not our children, impossibly high expectations, and when we exhaust ourselves trying to meet them, we swing the other way. We either drop all expectation in defeat, or we get mad and yell, and, feeling guilty about that, we grant a general amnesty on rules and regulations until we can no longer stand the chaos, and off we go, swinging back over to the other side. Once we find ourselves on this pendulum, it is nearly impossible to get off.

Parents who find themselves swinging back and forth and struggling to find a level of authority that feels comfortable may be tempted to idealize those who have the apparent self-discipline and inner conviction to remain at either pole. While many parents may not be entirely comfortable with the 'tiger' or 'free market' approaches, they admire the confidence of those who fully embody one or the other. Those who are constantly questioning themselves envy apparent lack of doubt.

But by treating the raising of children as a science and not as an art, both 'tiger' and 'free market' parents deny the fluid nature of children, of parenting and of family life. It is never a 'one size fits all' process. **The truth is, depending on the child and the context, there will be situations that absolutely call for the 'tiger' mom or the 'free market' mom, as well as times when a more middle-of-the-road approach is appropriate. The hard part – the hardest work – is in knowing what is needed when.** Without the luxury of a fixed formula to hide behind, it is much more likely that problems or mistakes might be traced – egads! – to you.

Making choices is the most challenging activity humans engage in, and it is one that requires us to bring together all of our capacities at their highest levels. Yes, at the bottom of it, both the 'tiger' mom and the 'free market' mom avoid making choices because they fear making mistakes, and because of that they have an uneasy, one-dimensional relationship with authority (and with their children).

The error that both the 'tiger' mom and the 'free market' mom make is in thinking that parental authority is concerned with who the child is – with the very being of the child – rather than with the child's behavior in the present moment. The 'tiger' mom wants to assure herself that her child will be someone of whom she approves, and so she controls everything her child does. The 'free market' mom fears doing anything that might somehow damage or influence her child's being, and so she does nothing to curb or guide her child's behavior. Both make the classic mistake of judging a child based on his behavior. It is true that a child's behavior is connected in some ways to who he is, but it is more a window than a reflection. We must be very careful about what we infer of a child's inner being from what he presents to us on the outside. The child and his behavior are not one and the same.

Consider this: what if our children were born with the seeds of all that comprises their being? Whether they are shy or outgoing, steadfast or flighty, talented with wood or a disaster with anything electronic, gentle with small children or a terror among anything refined – whether they are easygoing and cheerful or perpetually focused on what is missing and wrong, their basic temperament, personality and inclinations are all present, if not yet fully developed, right from the beginning. Their strengths and weaknesses, in a very rudimentary way, are part of their being from the very start. What if we knew – guaranteed – that our children would carry these seeds forever, no matter what we did or said?

When a challenge arises, would we feel more free? Would we be able to see our children more clearly, without the guilt screaming in our ear to fix them now, make them *be* different? Could we accept that they would always carry these aspects of their being in some way and feel free to simply deal with what they are *doing* right now? When the being is separated from the doing, there is so much less worry, so much less guilt. It is a whole different problem, one that is more manageable because it only exists in the moment. There is no worry about 'How can they get on in the world this way?' There is just 'What can I do right now to help them communicate more effectively, or be more considerate, or figure out this math problem?' You only have to worry about this moment, without the weight of a happy life in the balance.

In a fundamental way, our children already are who they will be. In the big questions, you are not irrelevant, but you are a supporting actor only, not the principle one. I am not trying to be flippant or oversimplify. Until, at least on some level, you can accept this, you will be caught, holding yourself responsible for that over which you have no control – who they *are* – and this leaves you powerless to guide where you do have an influence: what they *do*.

Sweating the Small Stuff

So much of the confusion and worry over authority comes from parents wondering how much is too much or too little. There is no fixed answer to this (sorry!), but it can be more helpful to ask not how much authority is necessary, but where it is most effectively directed. You may have heard the saying 'Don't sweat the small stuff.' Essentially, this means that you should not worry about the relatively minor difficulties but instead, put your limited time and energy towards the bigger questions and challenges. Sometimes this is referred to as 'picking your battles.' It is said that since we can't address every issue all at once, or even at all, we should pick the most important ones, the big ones.

But in parenting, this is exactly backwards because it focuses our energy where we have the least influence, as well as where it ultimately might not belong (who our children are), and directs it away from the areas where we have the most influence, and, as well, the most nourishing influence (what our children do).

The larger questions are not ours to answer: Will he be a leader, an entertainer, a teacher, an artist, a listener or a talker? Instead of aiming our authority and influence toward the end product, we would do better by putting our energy into the ground in which the seeds are planted.

That ground out of which the seeds that are our children will grow is, simply, their day-to-day life. Anti-climactic perhaps, but life is made up largely of the sum of little interactions and events, punctuated occasionally by big adventures, challenges and earth-shaking discoveries. Our children's character and their ability to express who they are, to put their best foot forward given who they are, is built in the spaces in between the big events. It develops in tiny increments by the inexorable accumulation of daily interactions. These lay down a surprisingly powerful foundation. How your child responds to great challenges, opportunities and setbacks once he is on his own depends on how he has learned to handle the most seemingly inconsequential moments at home. This is where your attention, your influence and your authority belong. **So, the bottom line: sweat the small stuff, and the rest will fall into place.**

What is the small stuff? That can only be fully answered by you, but I will suggest a minimum, a baseline from which to start and to which you might possibly add as you go: **manners and chores.** Learning to speak and act respectfully, even in challenging conditions – i.e. having good manners – is a way in which your child can affirm and be confident in who he is while he is among others, including those who are very different: something desperately needed in today's world. Household chores, those mundane, repetitive, always-needing-to-be-done tasks, provide fertile ground for the development of not just good habits, but your child's sense of self-worth and his awareness of how he fits into the fabric of life.

It is important to think about what matters to you most in your day-to-day life. If you are not clear about it to yourself, how can you be clear about it for your children? The following is my family's list, in order of importance:

1. Act kindly and respectfully to all;
2. Work hard;
3. Have fun.

These are our priorities, day in and day out. It turns out that this has been a pretty workable framework for us. It is applicable through all the stages of life (so far, anyway). It has allowed our children the freedom to express themselves and to explore a variety of avenues and sometimes even personas within basic guidelines which are immutable and are, therefore, utterly reliable. It has allowed my husband and me to feel confident in our insistence that there are certain lines concerning safety, respect and responsibility that must not be crossed. These are our expectations every day. We have very few hard and fast rules in our house, and they all stem from these. What are your priorities? What is your list?

What is Authority?

Ho Hum urges us to act with authority, but what is authority, after all? When we think of authority, often we have negative images: a rigid and demanding person in a position of real power, or an unresponsive, bureaucratic petty tyrant.

In the context of Ho Hum, authority is not punitive. It is not heavy-handed. It is not something to be endured. It is not the use (or abuse) of power, although the measured, confident and affirming hum of authority underlying your actions can carry tremendous power. Authority, as I'm using it here, means you bringing together your care and understanding and your wisdom and experience, along with your will to follow through with whatever action you determine is required. **Your authority is your higher self, your heart and mind and will coming together and carrying your whole family with it.**

You are not simply the captain of the ship; you are the ship. Your authority is the vehicle on which your children ride, buoying them along as they test out possibilities and variations. It is what carries them until they master their own stroke, delivering them to the place where they are ready to voluntarily disembark, first for short, exploratory trips and, before you know it, to travel their own way. No wonder we sometimes feel bent with exhaustion. We are literally carrying the weight of the world.

You already have authority, simply due to your life experience. We can always learn from our children. They teach us so much about love, about wonder, about the surprisingly vast array of giant excavating machines that can be seen on building sites if you stop and watch at every one you pass! And while we learn from our children in many ways more than they learn from us, they are entrusted to our care for a reason. Don't underestimate how much you have to teach them and how much they are hungry to learn from you. They need us to be the adults, to be the authority, to guide them so that they can come into their full being and flourish. We should not be afraid of our authority, nor should we take it lightly.

The Three Elements of Authority

The challenge with authority is to find balance. **There are three elements, or legs, upon which authority rests.** As with any three-legged stool, if one leg is overly long or short, the seat will be unstable. If any one leg is missing, the stool cannot support any weight, and the whole structure collapses. So it is with us parents. We must find the balance point between our minds, our hearts and our will.

The mind is the thinker, the planner, the one who determines the long-term goals and the more daily expectations. It holds up each challenge against a template of past experience. Our knowledge and understanding allow us to act instead of reacting and give us direction so that we are not merely blundering or blustering. The mind allows us to look through the lens of the world and see our children as the world sees them.

The heart is our emotional self, which keeps us abreast of the currents and ripples that our more logical mind might overlook. Our emotions are our feedback system. They tell us if our plan is working or if adjustments need to be made. Our heart allows us to act with warmth and love. It allows us to look at the world through our children's eyes. It allows us not only to accept, but embrace, the full being of our children.

Will or action is the third element. All the knowledge and love in the world will come to naught if we are unable to act upon it. Action is our connection to the world and the people in it. If our love and understanding are our inhalation, action is the exhalation, the follow-through. With the support of our minds and our hearts, we can respond with confidence, knowing that if the situation changes or if it becomes clear that something isn't right, we can adjust. We are not bound by any one parenting approach, but can choose according to the specific circumstances at hand. We are free.

Ho Hum teaches us that our authority is a given, and when balanced between the three supporting legs, it is a powerful, uplifting force. Like our emotions, we need to invite it in, learn to accept its presence and really become comfortable with it. It is a manifestation of all that we are and of all that we have to offer. Our children need this from us. They need to know, without any doubt, that we are in charge and that we are watching and will swoop in or step back when necessary. They need to feel the wisdom and the love that underlies the guidelines we set for them. They don't want to live in a world where things just 'work' or 'happen.' They want to see you there, with your big mother-spoon, stirring the pot.

There is a fourth element. It exists independently of the other three. Without it the structure and strength of your authority will stand, but this added element provides a cushion, something that makes it all a bit more comfortable. This last element is **humor**. It is the big needle that pokes the giant hot-air balloon of unrealistic expectations. It is a freight train making its inexorable way through the varied landscape of your life, carrying its cargo of truth. It is the middle of the pendulum swing, where we drag our feet along the ground, scuffing it and re-connecting to the reality, the gravity of earth, before we fly off again. Our troubles come from not seeing and not understanding what we see. Humor pulls away whatever veils we have constructed. That is why it is such a relief. And, it reminds us to find the joy in the storm.

Where to Start

Define your 'small stuff.' What are your priorities? We tend to think of qualities first, and that is a good place to start. Once you have a quality in mind – say, being responsible – think about what a responsible child *does*. Think in concrete terms: 'My child hangs up his bath towel,' instead of 'My child is responsible.' For now, it is enough to start working on shifting your focus from being to doing.

Chapter Three
Using Actions and Experiences Rather Than Words

Power Struggles

Imagine you are a senior employee at the State Department, and the White House has given you a special commission. You must find a person who can represent the nation's arguments in the face of powerful opposing interests, a person who will not cave in to the most professional persuasion of practiced diplomats or to the threats of internationally renowned thugs, a person who will hold to their own agenda no matter what comes. You salute the president, open the door and present your chosen representative... a four year old.

Anyone who has ever tried to win an argument with a four year old will know that this is no joke! Seriously, do you ever find yourself explaining to your child why something must happen after she has refused to do it, hoping to win her over with your earnestness and superior logic? Have you ever pressed your point by yelling or berating? When an outing is over, do you have to tell your child repeatedly that it is time to go, and still she refuses to come along? Have you ever bargained with your child, offering up a treat or reward in exchange for good behavior? Have you ever threatened your child with punishment if she does not stop misbehaving? Have you ever rationalized your child's misbehavior after being defeated in your efforts to stop it or redirect it? If you have, you would be in good company, sharing the dubious spotlight with the majority of other parents. I would be there, too.

These situations don't paint a particularly pretty picture. Certainly this is not how we imagined ourselves as parents. How is it then that we find ourselves in these power struggles? When we lose, we feel ashamed of our weakness, and when we win, we still feel like failures. We just want our children to listen to us. So why don't they? Why is it that we so often find ourselves sucked into arguments with them? Is there a better way?

That is what I was wondering, back when my daughter was four years old, and I was pregnant with my son. How could I discipline my child without crushing her spirit? I was determined to be a positive parent, one who did not order her children around, one who was sensitive to their needs, one who gently enlisted their cooperation to get things done, in short, one whose family lived in harmony with one another. So why did my husband and I find ourselves in long, drawn-out arguments with our small daughter? That was not part of the scenario I had in mind. Something, it seemed, was missing from the picture.

A power struggle boils down to a contest of wills. Someone will win, and someone will lose. Most parents sense rightly that this is, in fact, a no-win scenario. The 'tiger' mom fast-forwards past the struggle by making sure that the outcome is certain: she always wins. She disciplines her children with force, overpowering her children with her own will. The 'free market' mom avoids the struggle by expecting no discipline. She always loses. She believes that she is empowering her children by exerting no will of her own.

The unfortunate lesson that both of these mothers teach their children is that it is an either/or, win/lose proposition where there is room for only one winner. The rest of the mothers, whose approaches are somewhere between the two far ends of the spectrum, struggle on, as I did with my daughter, coaxing and suggesting and admittedly sometimes arguing, and wishing that it didn't have to be this way.

It doesn't. Harmony does exist. It is not a wild dream. The key is Ho Hum. It is just that errors in our understanding keep us from achieving it. One error is mistaking authority for power. Another error is mistaking words for action.

Let's face it. A certain amount of raising children involves getting them to do the things that we want them to do and stopping them from doing the things we don't want them to do, with periods in between when it doesn't really matter what they do. If we were honest, we would admit that we want them to want what we want. Then there would be no conflict, right?

We imagine that there might exist some sort of magic plane of synchronicity where all of our wants and needs miraculously dovetail together, and we think that if we were just relaxed enough or positive enough or creative enough or _____ (fill in the blank) enough, we could exist there, and we would never find ourselves in conflict with our children. What I didn't understand was that it is not the conflict that crushes our children's spirits. It is not making our kids wash the dishes, or the dog, or the car, or all three, that crushes them. What matters is how we do it.

The Difference between Power and Authority

I was reluctant to act using my authority because I mistook that for using power, for overpowering, and yet I knew that what I was expecting was not unreasonable. Power is the unfettered use of your will to control others. You do things because you want to and because you can, and there is no balancing effect from either knowledge and experience or love and understanding. Authority, on the other hand, is the foundation of Ho Hum and is balanced between thought, feeling and will. When you have authority, you are not in control of others so much as you are in control of yourself. You know what needs to be done, and you do it. **Power controls. Authority acts.**

Those parents who rely on power generally seek to avoid conflict or deny that it exists. Parents who rely on authority understand that conflict is inevitable, and they understand that its presence is not a sign of weakness or failure but is simply the reality of different beings learning to live among each other. For those who act with authority, *how* a conflict is handled matters most. They may not always welcome the conflict, but they recognize it and accept it – Ho Hum – as an opportunity to restore harmony. I had to learn that power struggles are not the inevitable outcome of conflict and that conflict is not a sign of failure. A conflict calls for Ho Hum. It calls for authority. It is a call to action.

Action, Not Words

Remember the three principles of Ho Hum:

1. Be calm;
2. Be confident in your parental authority;
3. Respond with action and experiences rather than words.

This chapter is about the third principle. It is about what goes wrong when we try to alter our children's behavior with talk alone. It shows how to break that habit and move to a more effective, positive mode in which we respond to behavior not with words but with actions and consequences. Children learn through experiences more than through verbal instruction, so we as parents need to figure out how to give them the former and reduce our dependence on explanations, scoldings and arguments.

Ho Hum calls for us to be calm. That means listening to and including your emotions but not being driven by them. It also means accepting the challenge of what is before you, and that means being willing to address whatever conflict or problem you and/or your child are experiencing, and *that* means acknowledging that you have the authority to do so. This is, after all, your job. Remember, all that emotion is telling you that this is important and that *you*, with all of your experience and understanding, are the chosen one for this job. It is time to focus, and it is time to act.

This is where most of us make another error. We mistake words for action. It feels wrong to yell at or threaten our children with punishment, so we assume that doing the opposite is the answer. We resolve to be relentlessly positive. We encourage. We explain. We praise. We are unerringly reasonable and kind and patient. We think that if we could just choose the right words, we could all share in the treasure of peace and harmony.

So, what is wrong with being positive? Nothing. It is just not a substitute for actions and experiences.

An example: A mom arrives at her friend's house, pulling her car up to the garage. Her children, aged three and six, are both belted into car seats in the back. Waving to her friend as she gets out of the car, Mom opens the back car door and reaches in to unbuckle the kids. Her upper half is bent in through the door for a long time. Eventually, she stands up with hands on her hips and breathes a big sigh of frustration. Then she ducks her head back into the car and speaks to the children in an urgent but reasonable voice. They won't get out of the car. She stands up again and looks at her friend with an embarrassed smile. The friend sympathizes with her predicament and asks if there is anything that she can do to help. 'No,' Mom says, and, painting an extra-chipper smile on her face, she tries another tactic, this time pointing out all of the temptations available in the yard: the swing set, the balls, and so on. No luck. The children won't budge.

The two women talk for a moment, but the children begin to fight. Mom, already vexed by their recalcitrance and her failure to get them out, grimaces and says, 'All right, we're going home.' She reaches back in to buckle their seatbelts and there is more wailing and fussing. Now, of course, the children want to get out and play. The older one pouts while the younger one cries. Mom apologizes for the scene. 'All right,' she sighs, and with whoops of joy, the children pile out of the car and rush to the swings. Later, when it is time to go, the children don't want to leave – no surprise there – and the whole scene plays out in reverse. 'Time to go!' Mom calls. The children ignore her. A paragon of patience, she lets them play a little longer. They are having such a good time. She hates to interrupt their play. But eventually, it really is time to go, so she tries again, explaining why they must go – lunch and other excitements are waiting at home, perhaps even a special dessert if they come along quickly. After considerable cajoling, and with a smile frozen onto her face, she manages to get them into the car.

Ouch. A difficult morning. While this mother's ability to maintain a level of equanimity throughout the whole scene was admirable and her ability to respond positively showed great self-control, it was, in the end, a power struggle, and one that she largely lost. If she had yelled or threatened, it is possible that she might have won the battle, but she didn't want to overpower them, to verbally beat them into submission. And she was right not to. But still, her positive words were no help either, and the morning was very stressful and unpleasant for her, and for her children, even though, on the surface, they appeared to get what they wanted.

She made a fundamental mistake, the same one that most parents make every day, the one which leads to power struggles: she mistook words for action and experiences. Words, whether they are positive or negative, will not open the door that leads through conflict to harmony. Words do have a place, a very important one, but when we rely on them instead of acting, those very words, even the positive ones, end up sabotaging us. Words are no substitute for action and experiences. The more you speak, the less you act.

By all means be as positive and encouraging to your children as you can, but **once you find yourself in conflict (meaning: your child is engaged in any of a million ways of saying 'no'), it is time to switch from speaking to acting. Yes, literally use as few words as possible. Your children need to experience change, not to be told what you need them to do. The more you speak, the less you act to transform their world.**

Parenting in Action

Part Three of this book contains many and various examples of effective parenting action and response, but a strong understanding of parenting action can be gained with the question: **If my child was imitating me, what would she be doing right now?** If you are arguing, debating, getting embroiled in long negotiations or indeed having a tantrum, your children are learning these behaviors from you – you are teaching them that these are the expected responses to a power struggle. Can you find a way to move from these verbal modes to modelling what it is you want your child to *do*?

If what your family needs is for you to be leaving the party, for example, then packing your things, handing your children their coats while putting on your own, and saying your farewells is going to be more effective than sitting on the sofa saying 'We really should be going now.' Acting rather than speaking means tidying alongside your children, rather than telling them to tidy up. It means getting up and leaving the café rather than threatening to leave the café. Action means lifting your screaming toddler out of the play car rather than trying to persuade her out.

Shifting from responding with words to a focus on your child's felt and lived experience also means retracting freedoms if they are not used responsibly, so she grasps the connection between greater licence and her own willingness to take on responsibility. It means calmly, consistently and kindly maintaining a consequence for difficult behavior, so your child learns through experience: 'Every time I behave this way, this is what happens.' It means finding ways for your children to put right their mistakes so that they can feel the shift from guilt to making amends.

Overall, this third principle of Ho Hum involves thinking about what your child is doing and experiencing and making changes there instead of using talk. Children will very rarely alter their behavior in response to being told to do so.

If we return to the mother whose children wouldn't get out of and then into the car, we see that she, as we have all done, consistently responded with words: patient, positive, tolerant, but ineffective words. Her children's experience was that when they whined and fussed and fought and refused, nothing much changed for them or in their world. They received words that washed over their heads, rather than change or actions that they could absorb. How different would their experience have been if their mother had calmly gotten back into the car and driven home? And had returned home in the same way from future outings if things went wrong again? This is a response that the children could have physically experienced. It would allow the three principles of Ho Hum to reinforce each other: it would have shifted Mom out of a mode of explaining, cajoling and arguing into a mode of action. It would have enabled her to step into her parental authority, making decisions on behalf of the family because she, unlike her children, understands the wider context and knows what visiting means. This active mode would also probably have made it easier for her to stay calm and acknowledge her own anger and frustration, rather than having to suppress these feelings under positive talk.

The Seven Deadly Non-actions

The following is a list of what I call the Seven Deadly Non-actions: explaining, repeating, yelling, asking, rewarding, threatening and rationalizing. These are the most common ways in which parents talk themselves into the quicksand of power struggles. By avoiding these and responding with action and experiences instead, you will find that you are more able to move forward.

1. Explaining.

Small children go through a period when they ask 'Why?' about nearly everything. The 'Why?' of a two or three year old is not a request for scientific explanations of natural phenomena; the child asks 'why' to express her wonder. If she is asking for an answer, it is not so much to the question of how or why the world works. She wants to know if the pattern of the world is complete, if all is well and good, and if, as part of that pattern, you love her.

During this time, the child's awareness of the world around her grows, and parents find their own sense of wonder renewed. Allow that wonder to reside in your heart without rushing to label, categorize and explain cause and effect. Let her love the world first, before she understands it. If the child does not receive the comfort that she seeks, she will continue to ask 'Why?' until the parent's patience is worn thin.

However, when a child asks 'Why?' at the moment we announce it is time to leave the playground, she is not expressing wonder, nor is she seeking information. She is expressing displeasure. She would rather stay and play. She has, no doubt, picked up quickly that asking 'Why?' or fussing are effective tools for diverting or delaying.

Rather than using the old and discredited 'Because I told you so' retort, we explain. We know that we are expecting our child to do something she doesn't want to do, and in order to soften the blow, we give her reasons. We think that this shows respect for her developing intelligence, that once she understands how reasonable we are, how logical and sensible we are, she will be swayed by the weight of our argument and will be willing to comply.

The theory sounds good, but unfortunately it has no basis in reality, which is why it rarely produces the hoped-for result. Children, while they have an innate and often delightful wisdom, do not operate out of logic. The child under seven takes in information through her body. She learns from what others do, and she processes that learning, internalizes it and makes sense of it, by imitating, by copying what others are doing. I am not saying that your child is not capable of thought or of being verbally intelligent. What I am saying is that before she is seven years old, thinking is not her primary way of engaging with the world.

When you explain something to your child, do you find that she jumps up and does what you ask, or do you find that most often she 'explains' back, or asks why? Explanations lead to arguments. **Unwittingly, by explaining, we are teaching our children to argue. We give reasons why, and they give us reasons why not, or vice versa. Two, three and four year olds argue because we model it for them. They are simply doing what they do best: imitating.**

The reality is that the reason your child has to leave the playground *is* because you say so. You say so not because you are arbitrarily and capriciously wielding power for the sake of power but because that is the way the world is. That is the pattern. You go to the playground, and then you leave the playground. Your child just doesn't know it yet.

She is only aware of her own tiny sphere of experience. How could she be expected to understand that there are other threads that must be woven into her day? There is a trip to the grocery store or the post office. An older sibling must be picked up at school. There is lunch to be made, eaten and cleared away, a nap and so on. She can't see the larger pattern yet. She does not have enough life experience to be able to step back, separate herself from her immediate activity, her immediate world, and put the pieces together. That is your job. You are the adult, the parent, the authority. You are the one who knows and understands. It is your job to help her weave her small piece of the world into the larger pattern.

So while you don't want to go back to saying 'Because I told you so,' you don't want to explain, either. **When you explain, you invite arguments and resistance.** The explanations don't help her understand the pattern. She learns how her own thread contributes to, supports and is supported by the greater pattern of life by *doing*. Explaining is a diversion from true action: for both of you. It only prolongs the time when you must, finally, act. It is far better to skip the explanations and inevitable arguments, and to go right ahead and act. In this case, since it is time to leave, you leave, collecting your child if need be, calmly, gently and firmly.

What I have learned through many intractable disputes when my daughter was four, which were ultimately frustrating for both of us, is that a parent insisting on an order to events is a comforting confirmation of authority for children, not an unfair assertion of power. In the case of leaving playgrounds, a wise mother is sensitive to her children's needs and understands the larger pattern, which means she doesn't act arbitrarily. She gives her children time enough to really play, but not so much that they become hungry and overtired. When she sees that her children are starting to show signs of needing a shift – they are no longer lost in play but are beginning to bicker, or they might have finished up on the swings and are wandering over to the sandbox – she acts. She doesn't let the moment slip through her fingers because her companion beside her on the bench is in the middle of a juicy story.

She is aware of the pattern, the greater rhythm, and so understands when the right moment to leave has arrived, and she has enough will and enough self-discipline to act when she recognizes that moment. That understanding, knowledge and will is her authority, and when her action is guided by that authority, it is ultimately a great comfort to her children.

2. Repeating.

Repeating yourself (also known as nagging) is the second Deadly Non-action. You are sitting on the bench at the playground, and you call out that it is time to go. Your child has found a friend and is reveling in the warmth of companionship: she and the friend both have on blue shorts, they each have a little brother, and look! they can swing forward and backward in perfect unison. Does she hear your call? Of course not. First of all, it is in her interest not to, and, in your child's defense, she is truly immersed in her delightful world of significant coincidences.

Ideally, you wouldn't call her the first time. Since she is so clearly involved with another playmate, you could walk over and speak to them both for a moment, acknowledge their bond: 'Look at you two swinging together! Anyone want one last push before we go? Yes? Here you go. OK, well, off we go. We'll look for you when we come next time.' And, waving to the new friend, you take your child's hand and you head off home.

Yes, it is fine to prattle on. It is not that all words are forbidden, and these words are validating and supporting the continuation of their bond. But it is not your words that draw your child away. It is your presence. The fact that you came over gives a sort of physical blessing to the act of leaving. Your child feels that she is worth your effort. Your physical presence carries her in a way that your voice cannot at this stage.

It is bad enough when our children ignore us the first time, but if we repeat ourselves, then we just reinforce the idea that what we say is worthy of disregard; that we don't, in fact, mean it. Repeating ourselves is *the biggest reason* why our children don't listen to us. Why won't they listen to us? Because we have trained them not to. It is as simple as that. **Repeating yourself encourages your child to ignore your words.** If you have called to your child that it is time to go, and she has not responded, calling again will not bring a better result. You will have to go to her and use your movement to jumpstart hers.

3. Yelling.

Yelling is the third Deadly Non-action that parents resort to when a child resists.

Sometimes fear is the catalyst: your child runs out into the road, and after you have hauled her to the curb, you let loose, venting your fear and hoping that the verbal assault will prove uncomfortable enough that she might think twice before doing it again. While the yelling in such circumstances is understandable, it is not particularly effective.

Fear sometimes precedes yelling, but the more common precursors are anger and frustration. You have called to your child over and over that it is time to go, and she is studiously ignoring you, or she moves farther off to be out of earshot. Alternatively (on a bad day: in addition), you have explained in a reasonable way why it is time to go, and your child has whined, argued or succumbed to total meltdown. In short, she is not coming. Patience is not the cure for the anger and frustration you feel (nor is it the answer to feeling embarrassed). Action is. Ho Hum: understanding, kindness, love... and action.

Yelling is an unconcealed attempt to overpower the child. Yelling can induce a child to comply, but while the parent may value the short-term effect, in the long term this kind of compliance will backfire. **We undermine our authority and damage trust when we yell.** If we do it often enough, we can cause real damage. We confirm to our child that all is *not* well with the universe, that we are *not* in fact bringing her into any sort of harmonious pattern or rhythm. Instead of modeling how to weave together the various needs of the moment, we shift the focus to ourselves. The child complies out of fear, but she has no sense of comfort from being part of the rhythm of the world. She feels exposed and vulnerable, and she does what she must in order to protect herself.

4. Asking.

Asking is the fourth Deadly Non-action. This is when we need to make a statement or give a simple instruction, but instead we ask a question. Here's a recent example: (I still do it. It is really hard to kick the habit.) Just the other day, after my son had vacuumed the house (his share of the weekly cleaning chores), I noticed the stairs were covered with huge wads of dog hair. I asked him, 'Thomas, did you vacuum the stairs?'

As soon as the words were out of my mouth, I knew how pointless they were. Either he did vacuum the stairs and he did a terrible job, or he skipped them. Either way, they needed to be done again, so instead of giving him the opportunity to be less than truthful, it would have been more comfortable for him and more direct if I had just let him know that the stairs needed his attention, briefly and without judgment. Simple statements work the best: 'Thomas: stairs.' Although in this instance I said: 'There is still enough dog hair on the stairs to stuff a couch.' He knew what that meant and took care of it.

At the playground, don't ask your child if she is ready to go when you really mean that it *is* time to go. **Don't confuse questions with statements.**

5. Rewarding.

Promising a reward for good behavior is the fifth Deadly Non-action. If the day has been glorious and you want to cap it off with an ice-cream cone, go for the ice-cream cone. It is fine to have a party to celebrate an extraordinary accomplishment. **It is not fine to motivate children to do the ordinary by promising a reward. It derails development of self-motivation, and teaches children to be selfish, to do what is needed only if there is an obvious, tangible, often material benefit.**

By rewarding children for the ordinary, we teach them that they are not truly part of the world like the rest of us mortals, but are somehow more special, more deserving, and ultimately, separate. They will try to soothe the discomfort of being separate by demanding more and greater rewards, none of which will leave them satisfied. The short-term pleasure is at the expense of long-term discomfort.

In addition to that grim sentence, when we offer rewards, we completely undermine our own authority. We are advertising that we lack confidence in it ourselves and are offering our instructions or requests with a bonus deal to make them an easier sell.

Rewards are also a false choice. Although your request is now framed as a choice (if you choose to leave the playground now you are also choosing an ice-cream cone), the child cannot actually refuse the reward and the request: she really is not free to choose to stay. This smacks of manipulation, which is the work of power, not authority.

6. Threatening.

Threatening is the flip side of rewarding and carries with it all of the same problems, except that instead of appealing to children's selfishness, instead of inflating them and making them feel they are above the rest, it elicits their sense of fear and makes them feel not more special, but invisible, diminished. As with yelling, threatening is connected to power, not authority.

Threats induce fear, which sabotages trust and undermines your authority. Don't threaten to leave the restaurant. Do it. If the consequence for throwing food is to remove the child's plate, then the proper action is not to threaten it, but to do it. Just remove it. Ho Hum.

7. Rationalizing.

Rationalizing, the last of the Seven Deadly Non-actions, is what we do when we give up or cave in. You have called to your child to let her know that it is time to leave the playground, or you have explained or threatened. You may have tried everything on the list, and still, she won't budge. You are tired, you don't want to create a scene. **If you haven't changed your mind, but are just caving in to resistance, be honest with yourself. Don't make the mistake of coming up with a 'reason' why it is better to stay than go.** This is 'rationalizing' – the 'boys will be boys' excuse, and it is never an excuse. If you are simply too tired to act, so be it. If you are going to let things go, do it and take responsibility for it, along with the consequences that follow.

Why Won't They Do *What I* Say?

An example: A family is out for dinner at a nice restaurant. The two small children are bored and decide to amuse themselves by playing with their straws and drinks. Mom, chuckling, admonishes them: 'Don't play with your soda.' She returns to her conversation, but the game is fun, so it continues and becomes more rambunctious. Frowning this time, Mom says, 'I really mean it. Stop it, or I'll take away your straws.'

The children freeze momentarily, one pouting and looking away, the other one smiling sheepishly, but once Mom stops glaring at them, they continue. The play evolves into a fight. One child has taken the other's straw and won't return it, so the other puts her fingers into the first one's glass, spilling it. 'OK,' says Mom, exasperated, 'that's enough.' The threat in her voice freezes the girls for a moment, but only for a moment.

The younger one comes over to her mother and slides into her lap, throwing a victorious glance over her shoulder at her sister. The older one, unable to gain access, tries another tactic and asks, 'Mommy, can I play with your phone?'

Mom, relieved that she has been presented with what she believes is a lifeline, grabs onto it. 'Sure,' she says. 'Both of you go sit there in the waiting area. But don't fight over the phone. And don't come back asking me to fix it for you. I don't want any more interruptions.' The girls scamper off with their prize. Mom sighs. Now she can finally relax.

But before you know it, the girls are back. 'Mom,' says the older girl, 'we can't figure out how to get the game to start over.' With a smile and a sigh of indulgent exasperation, Mom takes the phone and shows them what to do before sending them off again. She shakes her head and says, 'Why won't they listen to me?'

The children don't listen to their mother because she has trained them not to, because her words do not, in fact, have any meaning. She repeats, she threatens and she rationalizes. **No action or change flows from her words, so to her children, she is just nagging. They have learned to literally tune out her speech, treating it as useless and slightly annoying background noise.**

What the mother is really wondering is 'Why don't they *do* what I tell them?' If she wants her children to do or not do something, she must act. If she wants her children to listen to her, she needs to save her words for something that she wants them to *hear*, instead of using them for something that she wants them to *do*.

Have the Tantrum

Parents (like the mother in the restaurant) frequently rely on one of the Seven Deadly Non-actions because they are afraid that if they act, there will be an emotional scene.

An example: a mother is in the check-out line, and her toddler won't stay seated in the shopping cart. She explains why he needs to sit, she glares and repeats herself sternly, and she tells him that good boys who sit get stickers. Why doesn't she pick him up and set him down beside her? Because she is afraid that, by doing so, he will fuss and whine or, worse, throw a tantrum. In order to avoid the embarrassment of a scene, she sabotages her authority and reinforces for her son that what she says is not particularly relevant or important.

The truth is: you can't avoid the scene. If it doesn't happen now in the check-out line, it will happen later, and the longer you wait, the bigger and more frightening it will be.

So, go ahead: make a scene. It is far better to act to resolve a conflict and deal with any drama that results than it is to try to use one of the Seven Deadly Non-actions to avoid the conflict. Not everyone in the store or on the airplane will have dealt with a fussing toddler, but they have all *been* fussing toddlers. In order to respect the other people in the public space, it is worth moving yourself and your child out of the way, when possible, to manage the fuss. You don't want to make a spectacle of yourself, but neither do you want to sacrifice important lessons for your child on the altar of appearances. A 'Please excuse us' and a reasonable effort to step aside is all that is called for.

Modeling and Words

Listening, like speech, like action, is something we are constantly modeling for our children. Remember, they will do what we do. Do you listen to them when they have something important to say? If you are busy, do you let them know that what they have to say matters to you, and do you set a time later to sit down with them? Do you interrupt them when they speak? Do you jump in to argue or contradict? The power of imitation is always there, even if we are not aware of it. Very often, our children's listening skills reflect our own.

When we speak to small children, it is most effective to speak in images and to physically model what we want from them. Remember the whispered 'quiet as a mouse'? The whispering provides a model. The mouse provides an image. If you yell 'Don't shout!' you are modeling shouting. Small children will focus on your verbs: when you say 'Don't shout,' they hear 'shout.' If you are going to tell them what to do, stick to telling them what *to* do, and try not to tell them what *not* to do.

Actions not Words: Is it different with teenagers?

As your children approach their teen years, things change. Now there is an understatement! But you will find that the principles of Ho Hum apply at any age and at any stage.

No matter how old your children are when you read this, it is never too late to try Ho Hum. It is easier to start when your kids are young, but it can be done anytime. If you manage to replace talking with acting and experiences, you will be rewarded with a sense of rightness and harmony.

Notice, I don't say that you will have less conflict, although that may happen. Using Ho Hum allows you to deal with conflict in a way that is positive: positive, in the sense of being supportive, nourishing and effective – and positive in the sense of being sure. It feels right, not just to you, but to your children as well. Ho Hum doesn't make conflict disappear. Conflict is here to stay, but Ho Hum transforms it into a challenge that is manageable and a source of potential growth for both you and your child.

But you might be wondering whether the Seven Deadly Non-actions are still deadly when your children are older, when imitation is no longer their primary source of learning. In a word: mostly. Ho Hum always requires action, and talking is rarely a good substitute for it. **If you don't have a teenager yourself, believe me when I say that when conflicts arise, action and a focus on their experience is your lifeline. But that doesn't mean you should never talk to your kids.** It just means that when you are in conflict, talking becomes a dangerous and slippery slope. Less is more.

Is there a time when it is appropriate to explain things to your children or for them to discuss their wants and desires, to negotiate with you? Yes. As your children pass through the stages from early childhood to adolescence, you will be expanding the choices available to them. Yet your authority never diminishes. That would be equivalent to saying that your wisdom and experience diminish. (My husband is fond of Mark Twain's famous quote: 'When I was a boy of fourteen, my father was so ignorant I could hardly stand to have the old man around. But when I got to be twenty-one, I was astonished by how much he'd learned in seven years.') Children change, and so you will change how your respond to them, but only in response to their actual level of maturity. You don't give up authority as your child grows; she gains her own as she learns to temper her will and her emotion with her own knowledge and experience.

When your child approaches adolescence, she will again start to ask 'Why?' Or, more likely, 'Why can't I...?' On the face of it, the 'Why?' is simply a challenge to your authority. She is not interested in your reasons, she is interested in resistance or in changing your mind. But beneath that motivation lie the questions that the two and three year olds were asking: What is the pattern of the world *now*? Is it all well and good? How do I fit in it now? And do you *still* love me?

She rebels and challenges you because she mistakes authority for power, and she thinks that, like power, it is something that can be transferred. You have to show her, gently and with love, that the freedom and choice which she equates with power is actually something that comes hand in hand with maturity and responsibility – with her own emerging authority.

You can let your teenager know that you are open to hearing from her about anything – under certain conditions. **Negotiation has its place, but its place is not the middle of a heated conflict.** For example, I am open to my teenagers negotiating with me about what household chores they do or when they do them or how often, but I am not open to that discussion at chore time. Later, or before, they are welcome to present to me a respectful petition for a change, we can discuss it and I will consider it (and regardless of how awkward or tentative they are, when they are respectful, I will bend over backwards to find some way of saying 'Yes,' even if it is only to the smallest piece of it).

They have learned that challenging me doesn't bring the result that they wish for – not because I am a dictator, but because it is not my authority that is in question. It is theirs. When they show me that they have enough maturity and responsibility, when they can balance their wants with the needs of the situation, then I will consider more seriously and favorably their wishes for more flexibility on chores, for driving a car, for traveling alone, for whatever freedom it is that they are set on.

In teenage years, the answer to the questions underlying 'Why?' is: 'Yes, I absolutely love you, and the pattern of the world is not any different than before, but you are. Instead of being woven into it, you must take up the shuttle and begin to weave yourself in. I am here to help you when the threads get tangled. You don't have to push me aside but rather, you can join me here at the loom and we will see what you create. Look, I have been saving a spot for you.'

Words and Misinterpretation

One of the problems with words is that a lot gets lost in translation: interpretations of what we have said can vary, sometimes hugely. Like a game of telephone, what we whisper in our child's ear may be heard as an entirely different message, never more so than during adolescence.

An example: When our daughter was about thirteen, she worked for someone who did not respect personal boundaries. She wanted to handle it on her own, but it became clear that the situation was becoming more than uncomfortable. We sat down with Nina, and told her that, while we thought she was handling the situation in a mature and responsible way, we felt that her employer was dangerous, and we didn't want her to work there anymore.

Nina was incensed, so my husband, wise man that he is, thought to ask her to repeat back to us what we had said to her. She blurted out, 'You think I am no good at my job!' Far from it. We'd said we didn't trust the employer, but that is not what she heard. It is not that we were such poor communicators; it was just that she mixed what we said with what she expected to hear, what she feared hearing, what she felt about what she heard, and all the other aspects that go into a person's interpretation of words.

When it matters most that children hear and understand you, speak clearly by speaking as little as possible. And **when you have something important to convey, make sure that your actions and gestures show it, too.** If a picture is worth a thousand words, an action is worth a million.

Stories

Words in the right place *can* have tremendous power. For example, all people, and children especially, are nourished on a deep, soul level by stories. **Tell your children stories.** Read your children stories. Keep reading to them as they get older – all the way up to college and beyond if you can manage. Telling stories and reading aloud to your children is the single most effective way of developing their capacity to listen. And a story is the most natural vehicle for words and ideas.

The irony in this chapter is that I am writing to you in words, while saying that words have real limitations. I would rather be walking along with you, listening, laughing and commiserating and, most importantly for me, gesturing! You see, when I speak, I have to use my hands. My family once challenged me to sit on my hands and say something. I couldn't do it. Without my hands, there is no *emphasis*. Words just aren't enough.

Where to Start

Take a few moments to reflect on what you have said to your children in the last few hours or days. How much of it was truly worth being heard? How much of it was nagging? How much of it was a substitute for acting? Just notice for a while.

If you want to try using Ho Hum in your family, plan in advance. Think ahead to regular circumstances when you resort to using one of the Seven Deadlies and plan actions and experiences instead. Prepare what you will do, and prepare how you will respond if there is resistance.

Substituting action for words means breaking habits. The best way to do that is to substitute a good habit for a bad one. In Chapter Five, I will discuss family rhythm, which is the most effective way to establish good habits. But before we get there, Chapter Four covers choices: an important instance when actions are more effective than words.

Chapter Four
An Important Example of Ho Hum:
When to offer choices

Now that we have covered the principles of Ho Hum – staying calm, stepping into your parental authority, and using actions and experiences rather than words – in this final chapter of Part One, I want to address one of the most important, and most commonly misunderstood, circumstances in which we need Ho Hum. Offering choices to children is something that we parents routinely do, that indeed we often assume is a positive aspect of our parenting, expressing consideration for our children, showing flexibility and generosity. In fact, offering choices is a particularly problematic way of using words rather than acting. It is particularly problematic because it is an abdication of our parental authority, and as such it will likely undermine our children's sense of calm, thus leading to behaviors that undermine ours. Here is an important, practical and transformative way to put Ho Hum into practice: make choices and act rather than verbalizing questions and options for your children.

Whining and Choice

Few behaviors in children are more grating for parents, or more pervasive, than whining. Parents try everything from denial (it's just a stage, right?), to long and detailed explanations, to yelling in frustration. But whining is not a stage, it is a response. It will not spontaneously disappear when your children reach a certain age.

Children whine because they are given too many choices. Change this, and you can change their whining.

Here is a common scene: Mom arrives home with a box of pizza and her two little girls, Cheryl and Barbara, run upstairs to play. She calls to them, 'Girls, do you want some lunch?' The girls keep playing, and finally Mom goes to the bottom of the stairs and yells for them to come down. They do so, pouting, and sit on the sofa in the living room, arms crossed. Mom says in an encouraging voice, 'The pizza looks great. Do you want pepperoni or plain?' Cheryl whines, 'I don't want pizza.' Mom responds, 'Well, that is what we have. Do you want it on a plain plate or on the one with flowers?' Cheryl shakes her head and shouts, 'No!' Mom grabs two plates and doles out some pizza, putting it on the table. She says to Barbara, 'What do you want to drink? Milk?' Barbara says, 'I don't want milk. I want apple juice.' Mom says, 'Well, you have to have milk. Do you want it in a tall glass?' No answer. More pouting and arm-crossing. 'How about a straw? Would you like a straw?' asks Mom. Barbara bursts into tears, crying, 'I don't want milk.' Sorely tried by now, Mom loses her patience and yells, 'Stop that whining. Just sit down and eat your lunch!'

Observe a parent with a child sometime, or, better, observe yourself, and notice how many choices you offer your child over a day or even an hour. In the above scenario, Mom offers seven choices over a course of minutes. She is trying to encourage her daughters to participate willingly, to enable them to buy into her plan by giving them a choice, a stake in it. She is also hoping to avoid conflict and potential meltdown by diverting them with questions. **Contrary to popular belief, offering choices to young children is not an effective way to teach them how to make good choices. It *is* an effective way to encourage whining and invite power struggles.**

Offering choices is a prime example of parents – with all good intentions – using words rather than actions, avoiding their own parental authority and handing their rightful role over to their children, who do not yet have the capacities and life experience to manage what is being asked of them. The principles of Ho Hum tell us that another approach is possible for the Mom with the pizza, and is more likely to allow her to stay in tune with Cheryl and Barbara.

Were the choices Mom offered, the words she spoke, required?

CHAPTER FOUR: WHEN TO OFFER CHOICES

What would be lost if she accepted that she had, in her rightful capacity as Cheryl and Barbara's parent, already made the lunchtime decisions? Adopting Ho Hum, she could simply act from her parental authority: putting pizza on plates and pouring milk into cups. Mom can't force her children to eat lunch, but she can decide what is available and when.

The Trouble with Choice

It seems so simple, so innocuous, when we ask, 'What do you want?' We may think that we are asking about plain or pepperoni pizza, but we are communicating something else: by giving choices to our children, we are telling them that they are the point of reference and that what they want is of central importance. Instead of the focus being on the task at hand (eating lunch) the children and what they want have been catapulted to center stage, with Mom a captive audience waiting for their decision in order to proceed.

The trouble lies in the emphasis on the 'I' and the 'want.' We do our young children a disservice when we encourage them to be more self-conscious, more self-aware. To be able to make a choice, to be able to discern what 'I' want, one must be able to take a step back from the world and be separate from it. For children under seven, this is a stressful experience. To them, the world is all one.

Like a young player new to an orchestra, children flourish when they are carried by the swell of the music, when they get a feel for how their small part blends with the others, and when led by a conductor who has knowledge and understanding of the whole. Thrusting the novice to center stage for a solo leaves him entirely alone, without the guiding, supporting voices of the other instruments, and it at once shifts the focus from the mood and beauty of the music to his own performance.

Asking a child under seven to make a choice shatters his sense of being one with the world and encourages him to put an unhealthy focus on his own wants. There is a time for exploring one's sense of want, but childhood (under seven) is not it. A young child flourishes when the needs of the day are paramount – including his needs. Prematurely awakening a child's concern for his own *wants* without first establishing the supremacy of *need* leaves him vulnerable later to being ruled by wanting and unable to attend to the needs of a situation – to his responsibilities. The young child is best carried by the wisdom and experience of his parents and those who care for him. They are the ones who have the experience and understanding to know what is and what is not needed, and how to balance that with what he wants. It is their authority that is required.

Offering choices to adults is a sign of respect and a recognition of self-determination. For small children, feeling secure – being able to rely on adults to be responsible – is paramount over self-determination. A child who is given choices feels that sense of security shaken. By offering choices to a young child, we indicate that we are not in charge and are relying on him to take control. He whines to show his discomfort.

How many times have you heard a child say, when asked if he wants to wear his red or his grey t-shirt, that he wants to wear neither and, in fact, he wants something that is unavailable and he is unable to be satisfied no matter how many options the parent is willing to offer? **Choices rarely make small children happy.**

Two Kinds of Choices

There are two kinds of choices: conscious and unconscious. A child who goes to the closet and pulls out a building set is deciding to play. Every time he clicks one piece to another, he is making a choice: Which color to use? What shape? Where to put it? Children make these sorts of choices all day. They make these choices by doing. They are not consciously weighing options or considering possibilities and outcomes. They are not aware of being in state of wanting. They simply do things. The choice is not random, but it is not particularly conscious either. It is made primarily with the body.

It is a whole different story when the child's parent comes in and asks 'Do you want to play with your building set?' In this case, the child is being asked to make a choice based on what he wants and to bring what he wants to a level of awareness that he would never do naturally on his own. He is being asked to decide consciously. But he is unprepared for such decision-making.

Children can safely carry on making their own unconscious choices and learning from the results. Problems arise when parents *offer* choice, rather than stepping into their own authority and taking their own considered action.

So why do we do it? There are generally two reasons. First: we are trying to avoid conflicts with the associated whining and meltdowns (theirs and ours!), but, in fact, questions invite rather than avoid whining and meltdowns. And second: we have been led to believe that offering our children lots of choices will teach them how to make choices.

Teaching Children to Make Choices

Let's consider how we teach our children to make choices. Making choices – good choices – takes a lifetime to learn. It requires the highest-level capacities we have as humans. A child simply hasn't had time to develop those capacities, and, as discussed above, will rely upon what he does have when pressed to decide: a capacity to resist and to put his own desires first. Expecting your child to make a conscious choice before he is ready to do so is not fair to him, and is not teaching him how to make strong choices for himself.

The Child Under Age Seven

Children under seven learn through imitation. What you do and how you do it matters most. **During this time, it is really best to offer virtually no choices.** Your child is not ready to consciously make them himself, but he can lay the foundation for that by experiencing choice through your modeling. He does not have the capacity to determine whether a choice is a good one. You make the good choices, and he will learn what they are from your action. There is no need for explanations or any sort of 'lesson' about decision-making. Words will have very little impact.

Age Seven to Adolescence

The child from age seven to adolescence (around twelve to fourteen) learns primarily through his imagination. He needs to be able to create a story or an image and attach a feeling to that image to connect with it in some way. This is the time to start introducing choice in small and carefully applied doses. **Let him decide between two good or acceptable options (pepperoni or plain pizza; the red or the grey t-shirt), so that he can get a feel for it.** As he gets older, closer to adolescence, expand his range to who he invites over, or where you go out to dinner, or what extra-curricular activities to participate in. Just make sure that you are OK with all the options offered to him, so it is genuinely his choice.

He will be experiencing the consequences of his decisions as a feeling, not as a thought or an intellectual assessment. Take your time with this process. He is learning – from experience – about choosing. Give him choices where the outcomes are not unimportant, but they are not terribly heavy with consequence.

'Tweens' and Choice

Tweens may be ready to take on greater responsibilities, such as babysitting, mowing neighbors' lawns, or staying home unsupervised for short amounts of time. Their interests and initiative may emerge slowly and tenderly, or they may be bursting at the seams. Be mindful of hurrying the pre-adolescent. It's not appropriate to parent a twelve year old exactly as you would a six year old, but they are not ready for teenage life either. In today's world, tweens often dress and act like much older teenagers, but we must be careful to look beyond appearances and address the substance. It is tempting to substitute a cell phone for our guiding presence, but if your child isn't ready to do something without the cell-phone back-up, he is not ready with it, either. **When it comes to making choices, let tweens spend some time imagining what they would do, playing around with all the possibilities and outcomes of various decisions.** This is a great time to have lots of conversations with them: really develop the story of each option. 'What if...'

Teens and Choice

Between adolescence and adulthood (age twenty-one), your teenager is developing his intellect. He seeks truth and will learn best from those whom he can respect, those who are experts in their field. Don't be frightened off by the need for an expert. You are the perfect one to teach him how to make choices, since you have been making them, for better or worse, for a very long time. Now he is fully capable of thinking through the cause and effect of his own choices. He can think ahead and start to anticipate the outcome (although as we all know, just because teenagers *can* do this, doesn't mean they *will* do it!).

This is the time to let him make some choices that have real consequences. Let him experiment with choices involving 'how much.' How much time can he spend on Facebook and still get his homework done? How many hours can he work at his job and still have time for adequate sleep?

He will need to understand that freedom goes with responsibility: he will be given the freedom to make more choices as he shows that he can handle them. By expanding or contracting his freedoms in relation to his level of responsibility, he will get a good feel for that connection. Keeping him too close robs him of the opportunity to practice – and to make some mistakes – while he can still rely on you to help guide him and to let him fall but catch him before he hits too hard. Cutting him loose too early leaves him adrift. If you build his capacity with steady patience, when he has reached adulthood, he will have a solid foundation beneath him, and he will be ready to take the full responsibility for his choices on his own shoulders.

Where to Start

Giving choices to young children can be a hard habit to break, so begin by noticing when and where you offer your child choices. Recognize this as a way of speaking rather than acting, and as a stepping away from parental authority. Establishing a regular daily or weekly rhythm is a good substitute for those times when we tend to offer a lot of choices, and it is ultimately the most effective, but it also takes some time and effort to put into practice.

If you want to jump right in, pick one choice that you normally offer and... don't offer it. Act instead. Rather than asking your children what they want for lunch, make the choice yourself and proceed – prepare the PB&J and place it on the table without a word. Or, allow your child to act for himself by putting sandwich makings on the counter and letting him, with unconscious choices, put together his own sandwich. Here is Ho Hum in action: you are acting from your parental authority rather than speaking; you are modeling choosing for your children rather than expecting that an exchange of words will alter their behavior and move the day forward.

Part Two

Establishing Your Daily Environment:
The context for Ho Hum

Chapter Five
Rhythm: Giving time a pattern

In Part One we covered the three principals of Ho Hum: staying calm, being confident in your parental authority, and responding with actions rather than words. To help put this into practice in your own family, Part Two will look at how to establish an environment at home that uses and assists Ho Hum.

This chapter introduces rhythm, or how time and the form of the day can work for you when you are taking care of children.

Pre-emptive Action: Let rhythm do the talking

If words lead to power struggles, how are we going to get our children dressed, fed, packed up and out of the house in the morning? How are we going to move the day along? How can we get anything done if we are not going to tell our children what to do and when to do it? Inevitably, you will have to do some telling, but in order to keep that to the barest minimum, you can enlist the help of a powerful ally: rhythm. A rhythmic day and a rhythmic week can do a significant amount of the talking for you and will bypass many sources of conflict.

Rhythm is pre-emptive action. It contributes to family harmony by reducing the need to tell your child what to do and minimizing power struggles and resistance.

Rhythm is the combination of schedule and pace, with special attention paid to transitions. A schedule is just the order in which we do things, the structure of our day and our week. Usually, we build our schedule around main events. The timetable of the big ones – work, daycare or school – is often out of our hands. The rest is more under our control: sleeping, waking, eating, and any other activities that fill our day. Pace has to do with timing: how often we do something and how quickly we move from one event to another. Yet, having rhythm is more than having a schedule. A schedule alone is like a scaffold, external and rigid, while rhythm is more like your skeleton. It is a living structure that supports you and holds you within a certain range of movement – but is flexible as well. Rhythm is often compared to the breath: we breathe in and we breathe out. The pace may change according to the needs of our bodies, but the essential beat of alternating in and out is ever-present. Rhythm gives us more than the sum of its parts.

Some people are more comfortable with lots of structure to their day, others with less. When people think of having structure in a day, they most often think of it in terms of time and quantity: how many activities to schedule? How much structure is too much? How much is too little? They think of a day filled with structure as one in which every moment is mapped out. There is no free time, no down time. Some parents might nod in satisfaction at such an image, thinking that if their children are busy, there is less opportunity for them to get into trouble. Other parents might be horrified. With every moment scheduled, where is there room for the children to play freely, develop their imagination, dream?

Considering how much to schedule is important, but first I would like to encourage you to think not about the main events in your day and your week, but about the transitions between them. Think of transitions as a form of punctuation. If you have ever read a book out loud, imagine doing so without any of the punctuation – no pauses or periods, no question marks to make you reconsider. You would find yourself very quickly out of breath: you have lost that essential in-and-out pulse. Those periods and commas help to regulate our breath. There need to be moments to rest, collect oneself, and bring one part of the day to a close before turning to the next.

The Heart of Rhythm: Transitions

Attending to the *transitions* in your day is the key to establishing a strong and healthy rhythm. And yet, by their very nature, it is easy to overlook them. Then life becomes more challenging. For young children, the most stressful times of day are times of transition, when they move from one activity or space to another. These are the times when they need us the most. One of the paradoxes of a rhythmic household is that if we commit a little more time and conscious attention to these moments, they will ultimately take less time. **Truthfully, when considering adding an activity, the question to ask yourself is not whether you have time for the activity, but whether you have time for the transition before and after the activity. What children experience and learn getting to an event is often more important than what they learn from being at the event.**

How Many Events?

A rule of thumb: the smaller the child, the stronger the rhythm and the slower the pace. The mantra for young ones: less is more. The rest of their lives will be busy, busy, busy. Wait as long as you can before loading them up with activities. Even when they are teenagers with days chock-full of school, work, friends, sports, and so on, they will still need strong rhythm, but they can handle a busier schedule and a faster pace. Hopefully they will be managing most transitions on their own by then, but it is still worth observing some daily moments of collective pause, when everyone stops to take a breath together.

The other day as I sat writing this, my husband was talking loudly on the phone, and I was cooking dinner, answering my teenage son's questions about an essay and texting little murmurs of encouragement to my daughter who was at college with a bout of mononucleosis. Nobody was paying full attention to anyone. It was fairly chaotic, but part of what held it all together was that everyone in the household knew there would be a pause at dinner, a moment when we would sit together, catch our breath, share our thanks for the meal and each other, and really see and listen to each other. Afterwards we would clean up together, and then off we would go again.

An informal survey of the articles from *The New Scientist*, which my husband reads and quotes from, indicates that the most sure-fire way to help your children become good students and all-around, well-balanced individuals is to do two things: eat dinner together and ensure a good night's sleep. That's the power of rhythm. Lay that foundation as early as you can and keep with it.

A lack of rhythm is often the hidden source of tenacious problems. It is worth any effort to establish and strengthen your family's rhythm.

Evaluating Your Rhythm

It can be a sobering but illuminating exercise to take an average day and notice your transitions. You may have an already obvious trouble spot. For example, it might take half an hour and a day's allotment of energy and tears – theirs and yours – to get your kids dressed in the morning. Or perhaps leaving the house is a source of stress, with your reminders to get ready falling on deaf ears and resulting in a distinct lack of mobilization. That, combined with breakfast dishes left on the table, missing backpacks and forgotten shin guards (again!?), is enough to make the most well-balanced, kind-hearted mother feel like a harpy. Yes, but before you zero in on smoothing that one transition, it will help to look at your whole day – first, so that you can get a sense of the patterns and habits you have and can discern what is working and what it not, and second, because the most obvious trouble spot may not be the best place to start making changes. If you have an area crying for attention, notice that, but notice the rest, too.

So, first thing, observe yourself and your children for a day. If you are inclined, it can be useful to make a list or draw a map of the stages and events in your day. Keeping track of it in your head is acceptable but not ideal because you want to include as many details as possible without attaching any particular weight to them, and we tend to remember things by ranking them. No detail is too insignificant. The most striking ones may not be the most relevant.

Start by noticing the main events or the overall structure of your day. At the very minimum, that would include waking, breakfast, lunch, dinner and going to bed. What else happens? Start to fill in the gaps. Do you leave the house for work, school, errands, outside lessons or other activities? Is there a nap, a bath, a time for chores? Are there times that are not scheduled, when your child is free to play or just lounge around? When you have noted those down, ask yourself what happens in between *those* moments. If the kids have been playing outside and lunch is ready, how do they get from hanging upside down on the monkey bars to sitting before a plate with a peanut butter and jelly sandwich on it?

Keep adding in detail. It is easy enough to say, 'Oh, after their bath, they go to bed.' It is the lack of attention to the moments between those two events that can lead to so many power struggles, so don't turn away now, just as you are getting to the crux of it. If you are overwhelmed by looking at a whole day, pick one part: the morning or the evening. The most important thing is to go deeply into the transition and pick it apart, to get to the actual steps, one after another, that happen, or that don't happen!

As you fill in your map or your list or your memory, ask yourself the following questions about the events of your day and the transitions between them. Keep in mind that there is no right or wrong answer – you are noticing, not evaluating. Looking provides valuable information, and judgment only closes off our access to it.

* Who decides what to do and when to do it?
* How do you know when it is time to start/end an activity? Who or what initiates the transitions? How is that done?
* What do you say during the transition? Do you use any of the Seven Deadly Non-actions? (Are you judging yourself right now? Just note down your judgment and keep going. I have used them all at one time or another, so if you have used any of them, then you are in the same boat as I am, and we can consider ourselves in good company. Carry on.)
* What do you do during the transition to move things along? What else do you do? Are you on the phone or the computer, making dinner or folding laundry?
* What distracts you during the transition? What are you thinking about? Where is your focus?

* Are you judging your child or yourself during the transition? Does that make you feel or act differently?
* How do you feel before, during and after the transition? Do you look forward to transitions or do you dread them?
* How does your child feel? How does she respond to what you do and say?

Once you have spent some time noticing, go back and see if you can find any patterns. Some people get hung up first thing in the morning, but once they get rolling things go pretty smoothly. Others are great at getting something started but have a hard time wrapping up and moving on. Still others will find that nearly every transition ends in a power struggle. This is the time to do a bit of evaluating – but only about what works and what doesn't.

Ho Hum guides us to respond to the reality that is before us, but in order to respond, we must first know what that reality is, and that can be surprisingly difficult for us humans to nail down. Not only must we be calm – recognizing, accepting and listening to our emotions – but we must focus. As best as you can, set judgment aside and look, and if that is simply impossible, notice the judgments too and write them along with your other observations.

Acknowledge any feelings of frustration, anger, guilt, upset, despair, and know that what your feelings are telling you is that this is important. They are calling for your attention. Ho Hum also tells you to act: to determine what needs to be done based on what you see, what you feel and what you know, and then, finally, to do it.

Watch out for blaming. If you discover, or even if you knew all along, that your transitions are a weak spot, you may be sorely tempted to blame someone (your kids, yourself or your spouse are the usual suspects, but others can stand in as well). Blame is a time-honored method of avoidance. We all do it, so don't blame yourself for blaming! Regardless of how or why the transitions fell apart, you are the one who is going to put them together again. Blame is beside the point.

Rhythm is not a drill sergeant but a relief. If your days are hectic or tightly scheduled, a strong, smooth transition between waking and breakfast or between school and soccer can serve as a respite, a moment to catch your breath. If you have long, lazy days with few scheduled events, transitions serve as a predictable anchor, a time to collect scattered pieces. No matter what your parenting style is and how much structure there is in your day, children need strong and rhythmic transitions. This is non-negotiable.

Having smooth transitions lends an overarching coherence to the day, and allows children to sink into their activity. Rhythm lets them know when to attend to a task, but it also lets them know when they are done.

The Three Elements of Rhythm

You can make your transitions less stressful and more rhythmic and supportive by combining some imagination with the three basic elements which create rhythm: your clear presence; a predictable pattern of actions; and the use of song, story or verse instead of the Seven Deadly Non-actions.

Your Clear Presence

If we couldn't plan a day's meals while changing a diaper, or talk to a friend on the phone while cooking dinner and folding laundry, we would have to stay up to the wee hours just to get it all done (and we may have to even so). For parents, especially mothers, multitasking is a valuable skill and a way of coping with the never-ending waves of 'things to do' that wash up on our shores every day. Whether or not you have an outside job, you are working – and working hard, all the time.

Multitasking can lend some efficiency to what you do, but it comes at a price. If you are doing one thing (or more!) and thinking about another, you are not fully present with either. There are real benefits to be gained from letting yourself fully experience, without distractions, the job of, say, raking leaves: there is the screeing sound of the rake, the smell of the rotting debris, and the feel of a slight breeze on your neck, but oh! – now it is gone and you are alert for its refreshing return. You notice what your neighbors are doing and which hole in the wall the chipmunks favor. You are not simply getting it done. You are connected; you can feel the rhythm of the earth, and it carries you, and while you may be physically tired by your task, you come away with renewed inner strength and a sense of clarity and purpose.

This feeling of being supported and nourished even while making considerable effort is what your child wants and needs during the transitions in her day.

Now, you might say that not every moment calls for such attention: you are more than happy not to fully experience the moment when you are hunched over the side of the tub scrubbing the rust stains from around the drain. You might be surprised at what you could gain from doing so, but no, you don't have to be fully present all the time with everything, nor is it possible to be so.

But if you are having trouble with your children – and I mean *any* trouble – the first thing to do is to strengthen your rhythm, and that means attending to your transitions. And that means giving *those* moments your undivided attention. Your single-minded focus is the most powerful tool you have.

Rhythmic transitions are not random. Once they are happening, your child or an outside observer might not realize that you are, in fact, the conductor. They may not realize that the transition is tightly choreographed and expertly orchestrated because it flows so seamlessly. It seems so, well, obvious, just as the sun rises in the morning and sets in the evening. We go to the playground and then we leave the playground. We clean up dinner and head to the bath. We get dressed, feed the dog and sit down to breakfast. Or whatever. You may draw inspiration from the natural tendencies of your children, but you are the one who feels out how to synchronize those with the day's imperatives. You are the one, Ho Hum, who creates the pattern, the rhythm, the wave or current that will lift and carry your child.

Your clear presence is a potent, non-verbal call to your child to come join in. (Haven't you noticed that when you are deeply engrossed in something, it becomes irresistible to your child?) You, with your clarity and sense of purpose, draw your child in to be carried by the steady pulse of the day. For a few moments, you help her align the pattern of her own individual world with that of the broader one. She feels connected, supported, nourished, and revitalized. But in order for her to feel it, you must feel it. Even if the rest of the day is going to be one stressed-out marathon, during this one moment there is only getting dressed or leaving the playground or bathing or going to sleep. Be clear, be present, and breathe deeply. That is your baseline, your fallback position, your refuge and your best guide.

Inherent in that presence of yours is the clarity of your authority. You are the one who must decide what will happen and when. Your decision is not arbitrary. It is ever-mindful of each of your children, but it is not based solely on what they want, nor is it based primarily on what you want. It reflects the overall need of the family as a whole. If you seek to always accommodate your child's wants, you will not only find that you have become a servant to a selfish and demanding dictator, but you will find that your child is rarely satisfied with your efforts.

A Predictable Pattern of Actions

Transitions are all about change, and all changes, even the good ones, are stressful, especially for children. We adults can generally handle the adjustments involved in getting ready in the morning or finishing up a project and moving on to get dinner ready. We have had lots of practice. Small children face the transitions in their day as if each one were new and momentous because, to them, they are. When a child wakes up, she is not, as you might be, thinking ahead. She is engrossed in the immediate moment, whether that involves playing quietly on her bed, seeking out some breakfast to satisfy the rumbling in her stomach, or engaging in an ongoing battle with her brother over the stuffed dinosaurs. For her to stop doing that and do something else – say, get dressed – requires an adjustment, a shift in her focus and energy.

While expecting her to get dressed is not unreasonable, you will need to help her make that adjustment. She needs practice. Not only does she need to literally learn how to get dressed – put her legs through the leg-holes in her pants – she needs to learn how to shift her focus to getting dressed. Making that shift is a skill like any other, and skills are learned with practice and repetition. **When there is a regular pattern of events during a transition, the child learns the pattern deeply and physically, and she feels relieved and satisfied**

by the repetition of that pattern. Young children learn through their bodies by imitating the actions of those around them. They watch what others do and copy it. It is your job to model a predictable sequence of actions at the transition points of the day, which your child can imitate, over and over and over.

Children not only need repetition; they thrive on it. *You* may be bored by stopping every afternoon to see the same ducks on the way home from school, but your child is not. *You* may be tired of peanut butter and apple slices every day for an afternoon snack, but your child is not. *You* may want to read a different story every night before bed, but your child, up to about age eight, will be delighted to hear the same one, over and over again – so make sure you pick stories that you like! I believe my husband read *Fantastic Mr Fox* in its entirety each night for about a hundred nights running and never tired of it. Now that is great literature! Each family has its own favorites, and your child will end up memorizing the stories so that if you try to skip a part in order to hurry things along, there will be cries of outrage: a human rights violation!

That memorization, that wholesale ownership of the story, is what we are aiming for in our transitions. Like their beloved stories, we want our children to know, to anticipate with absolute certainty, what is going to happen first and what will follow during every transition. Your children will learn the motions so deeply that they are part of their muscle memory. Then they will do them without conscious thought and without constant reminders. Those familiar sequences, those habits, can be an emotional safety net during times of family stress.

Strong rhythm allows, indeed makes more exciting, occasional days of difference. On a day when we couldn't stand being homebound by a storm for another minute, we would throw a big blanket over the table and have a picnic underneath, with flashlights and stuffed animals and the dog, too – until she stole too many unguarded sandwiches. It was that much more of a vacation because of its delicious departure from the normal lunch routine. But having every lunch under the table, or scattered willy-nilly, as you please? No.

For those of you who prefer to fly by the seat of your pants, that is all well and good. Your day can be as spontaneous as you like (having free, unscheduled time is a rare luxury now, but everyone needs it, especially younger children, and even those busy teenagers), but make sure that there is some sort of punctuation, some reliable pause, or you may find that your child will melt down or fly into a rage unexpectedly. And if you find that your child does this during the one rhythmic transition that you have managed to establish, don't misinterpret that as a sign that the transition is the problem. It is the only time when she feels safe enough to fall apart. She is telling you that she needs more, not less, routine and pattern.

Just as you would move on from *Goodnight Moon* to other stories at bedtime, your transitions will also change over time. Remember that it is your presence and your actions that remain the catalyst. They get things rolling. But there will come a time when you don't have to go with your child to find her backpack, or go through the list of what she needs to bring. (This involves learning that when one looks, one has to actually search for the objects with one's *eyes*. This seems to be particularly difficult for boys.) You won't have to help her dig through the pile in the closet for the missing mitten or be there while she puts on her jacket. There will be a time when all you need to do is get your own bag together and jacket on and meet her at the car. Before you know it, if you want to think about the hair-raising implications of progress, she will be driving off herself, with or without her backpack.

So what do you do during transitions? What is the right way to get up, get out the door, get out of the pool or get to bed? What is the right pattern of actions? As you might have guessed, there is no one right pattern. Transitions are like Thanksgiving dinner. The main course is pretty much the same for nearly everyone except the radicals, but the side dishes vary a lot from household to household. The unspoken but universally understood rule, however, is that tradition trumps innovation: within each family, their particular menu is sacred and is not to be messed with. If you have cornbread stuffing and creamed turnips, you have cornbread stuffing and creamed turnips every time. It is the same with your transitions. What works for you may vary from what works for someone else, but the key is that you stick with your plan. That is what makes the transition rhythmic: it is utterly reliable – boring even, but only to you.

When our daughter was born, my husband wanted to have something special that only he did with her, just as I was the only one who breastfed her. He became the bather-in-chief. I butted out completely (well, at first I hovered, but I soon learned that sharing meant, shockingly, that he got to make his own mistakes, just as I got to make mine). Anyway, when she was about two years old, my husband went away for a few days, and I had to give my daughter her bath. Immediately I was told, 'Daddy doesn't do it that way.' I was clearly not sticking to the usual program, and while we managed to get the job done, my daughter stoically putting up with my obvious ineptitude, everyone was relieved when Dad got back to do it right. Maybe he started with her toes and worked up from there, or wrapped her in her towel just so. I have no idea, but she did, and that is what mattered.

Silliness can be a welcome part of your routine. Another part of our bedtime transition involved my children pulling the covers over their heads when it was time for my husband to come in and give them a kiss and read to them. He would 'sit' on the bed and wonder loudly, 'Where, for heaven's sake, might Nina or Thomas be?' and he would then proceed to 'lie' down to wait for them, complaining all the while about the 'big lump' in the bed, from which maniacal giggling could be heard. There was nothing particularly special about our night-time routine, but the fact that it was *our* routine made it special to us.

Reverence has a place in transitions as well, the most common being a time for saying grace before meals and before bed. In our fast-paced and scattered lives, it is worthwhile to take a moment to stop in silence, to hold hands quietly or light a candle, to be grateful for each other and the meal, a symbol of all that is good in the world. Mealtimes are often the only time a family has when all are present and not consumed with media and getting things done. A moment's pause to recognize and honor the nourishment received from both food and family will fortify everyone present, the children most especially. They have a natural feeling of awe and wonder for the world, and it feels right to them that something so familiar and daily be treated as the special moment that it is. For them, the presence of their family together, something so obvious that it is mostly taken for granted by adults, is deeply satisfying.

Going to bed is the polar opposite of a family gathered together to share a meal. It is a time of separation, when, for many children, they must enter the world of sleep alone. For the young child, the almost ritualistic bedtime routine is a reminder to her of how much she is woven into the fabric of the family. A bath, the hugs and cuddling are a physical embrace. The stories wrap her in the sound of a beloved voice, while at the same time they remove her from the immediate world, allowing her imagination to aid her in slipping out to the land of sleep. A lullaby does the same, with even less stimulus (another reason to repeat the night-time story – so your child is not actually awakened by something new and exciting). A prayer or short verse evokes protection, even if it is only the silly 'Good night, don't let the bedbugs bite!' that my grandmother used to say.

Use Song, Story or Verse

If you think of your transition as a form of punctuation for your day, you will get a sense that all transitions involve a connection of some kind between a leaving or closure of one thing and a beginning or opening of another. Your action is what calls attention to the mark on the page. The emotional tone determines whether there is just a comma – a whiff of a pause or a gentle change of direction – or a period – a full stop, where the activity is brought to a complete close, toys are rounded up and put away before moving on to what comes next.

Ideally during a transition, what you say is an extension of your action. It becomes part of the emotional gesture, adding warmth that lifts the child and sparks her imagination in a way that helps to carry her. It is tempting to initiate transitions with announcements and reminders: 'Time for lunch,' or 'Don't forget to brush your teeth.' While these don't have the immediate negative effects that the Seven Deadly Non-actions have, they lack any sort of galvanizing quality, and the fairly predictable lack of response from your child can leave you tempted to say more. Instead, let your words play a supporting role. Act first, even if it is only a leap up from the sofa with a loud clapping and eager rubbing together of your hands before saying, 'Lunch!' Let your action be the bulk of what you communicate, and let your words color it, adding flavor or emotional tone.

If the job of your words is to enhance your actions and to make them more inviting and compelling, announcements and reminders simply fall flat. They have little power to connect. In fact, they serve as more of a challenge, calling attention to the space between you and your child. What sorts of words help to bridge that space? What can you say that will draw your child to you so that together you can sail through the waters of change?

Compare these two approaches to leaving the playground:

1. Mom calls to her son, who is busy in the sandbox with a few other children, 'Time to go!' Her son keeps on playing, so Mom decides to give him a few more minutes and returns to her conversation. Distracted by that, she doesn't notice her son when he looks over to see if she is getting ready to go. She isn't, so he takes his cue from her and keeps on digging. A few minutes later, Mom tries again, a bit exasperated this time, 'Joshua, it is time to go. Really. We have all sorts of errands to do on the way home. Now let's go.' But Joshua is defiant now, so she marches over with hands on her hips and tells him to pack up his buckets. Arguments follow, ending with Mom stalking off and Joshua following, jaw set and tears in his eyes.

2. Mom heads over to the sandbox where her son is engrossed in digging. She is humming the same song she always hums when it is time to go. 'Is it time to go already?' asks Joshua, looking up dreamily. Mom smiles and nods her head. 'Here,' she says, 'go ahead and take a moment to fill that hole. I'll start collecting shovels. Is this our bucket?' Mom collects the toys while also saying goodbye to the other children in the sandbox. Joshua mounds some sand over his last hole and holds out his shovel to Mom, who hands him a bucket to carry. He takes her hand, and they head for the parking lot. 'To market, to market to buy a fat pig,' says Mom. 'Home again, home again, jiggety-jig,' replies Joshua, swinging his bucket.

In the first scenario, Mom expects to motivate her son with words and words alone, and when that doesn't work, she resorts to using the Seven Deadly Non-actions, repeating and explaining. The result is a power struggle, and as we know, everyone loses in a power struggle. Not only is this particular afternoon an unhappy one for both, but it lays the groundwork for future struggles. Next time, Mom will be expecting defiance and resistance and will either try to be more forceful, opening right up with yelling and threatening – which will likely be met with increased defiance from her son – or she will try the other tack and be obsequious, asking, bargaining, and finally rationalizing when her son holds his ground.

In the second scenario, Mom acts first by coming over. Her physical presence lends some gravity. She also hums a familiar 'leaving song,' which gently nudges its way into the depths of the world of play in which Joshua is engrossed. He can surface slowly, instead of being suddenly wrenched away. She gives him a moment to find a comfortable stopping place while she begins to collect the other toys. This acknowledges that he is still in the middle, but it also guides him to find an end.

Instead of telling Joshua what to say to the other children, Mom models the leave-taking, saying goodbye for him until he can do it himself. This also signals that it is, in fact, time to go. She gives him a bucket and takes his hand. On the way to the car, they recite their leaving verse: a snippet of a nursery rhyme. Each knows his or her lines, and the 'call and response' effect of it serves to connect them in their common purpose. Instead of being a brick wall, she is his bridge. The emotional tone is not one of breaking away but of continued belonging. It *is* hard to go, but it is much easier and safer to go when one feels that one is also arriving somewhere warm and welcoming. Mom gives herself and her son time enough so that the transition is not hurried and forced, but she is also clear that they will be going.

Using song, story or verse can lend support to transitions, and they are great substitutes for explanations and admonishments. Song engages children very differently than speech. It reaches past their conscious will and connects with their inner sense of rhythm. They become aware of their will in the context of that rhythm and naturally find a way to synchronize themselves with it. Singing just doesn't bring out resistance the way telling does. Verses are the same. If you use the same verses for the same transitions, they become satisfying, shared confirmations that all is well with the world – that the pattern, while changing, is familiar. Frankly, the use of song and verse is also of value because it gives parents something to say that is not one of the Seven Deadlies! It is so hard to break that habit, and singing, humming or reciting a rhyme or verse can literally keep your mouth busy with a better alternative.

Appealing to your children's imaginations with stories is another way to engage them in a transition. The logic of action is comprehensible to children, where a logical argument is only so many words to them. An image or a story, however, is even more up their alley. When the kitchen is transformed into a ship's galley, and your children must bring the grub out to the rest of the pirates, preparing the same old lunch takes on a whole new meaning. The children will be much more enthusiastic about participating in the regular lunch chores (although, as pirates, they may balk at washing their hands: totally out of character). Or something less involved: your child asks why she has to go to bed, and you say, 'Even the sun goes to bed.'

Stories and images can add spice, they can reassure, they can explain without explaining by creating a picture in words a young child can understand and relate to. The potential is endless, and I encourage even the most reluctant of you to try to stretch your own imagination and see what you can come up with. One aside: don't feel that you need to turn every transition into a story. The idea is not to entertain or make each one a new adventure. The transitions serve best by being the same thing most of the time, like the bland comfort food we all crave. But a story or image can be helpful in setting a tone or getting past a rough spot.

What Is At Stake for Your Child?

There is an almost symbolic aspect to transitions. On the surface they are just the progression of steps that we take to wake our children or get them ready for school, but they are much more than that as well. So that you can better understand what is emotionally at stake for your child at these times, ask yourself the following questions:

* What world does she inhabit now and what world must she move into?
* What is changing: place, activity, people?
* What is ending? What is beginning?
* Does the transition require an increase of energy, a gearing up and harnessing of energy in order to focus it on a task, or does it require more settling, a collection of what is scattered?
* What might she worry about or fear?

❋ What might she resist?
❋ What does she need to know?

A transition is comprised of a physical shift of some kind, getting out of the pool and going home, for example, but there is an emotional shift that must happen as well. **When you mesh the physical change in a way that supports the emotional change, you will have yourself a rhythmic transition.** Remembering that a young child's primary language is in the movement of the body, think first about what you and she can *do* during the transition. Ask yourself these revealing questions:

❋ Am I modeling what I want my child to do during the transition?
❋ If she were to imitate me, what would she be doing?

What might that mean at the pool? You might have to get in with her and play around for a few minutes. One, your presence in the watery world becomes the continuity she needs for leaving it. Two, when it is time to go, you can swim over to the side with her, helping her out as you get out, instead of standing impotently at the side, yelling at her or backpedaling once she has ignored your entreaties: 'OK, one more dive and then we really have to go.'

If you want your child to wash her hands after using the toilet, instead of asking her if she did it when she emerges, hand her the soap when she is done and wash your hands while she washes hers. If you want your child to put on her boots and mittens, instead of telling her to get ready to go while you are throwing another load of laundry in the washer or sending a last email, be heading to the door and putting on your own boots and mittens.

Will you always have to do everything with her? No. Once she has her part down, once she knows it backwards and forwards, you can let her do it on her own, just as long as you continue to do your part. There will be a time when a wave is enough to get her out of the pool, the sound of you rattling dishes on the stove will bring her to the kitchen to set the table, and she will wake up and get herself off to school without you. Her willing participation in the regular routine of the transition is one signal that she is ready for you to step back, but don't jump the gun. A more reliable signal comes when she lets you know that she has got it. She sees you get up at the playground and shouts, 'I'm coming!'

Put your time and effort in early. Lay a solid foundation from the start, and you will find that your transitions can be more than hassle-free: they can affirm and replenish the wellbeing of each individual and your family as a whole. That feeling of wellbeing will reverberate throughout your day, giving it a healthy flush. Your children will be grateful, cheerful and capable. If, for example, you fall ill, not only do they know how to take care of their part of the routine, but they know how to do yours, and they will be proud to show you that they can. If you are exhausted by a particularly long or difficult day, when you sit down heavily at the dinner table with a deep sigh, your children will reach for your hands and give the thanks.

I cannot emphasize enough that the key to rhythmic transitions is in the doing: the action. There is no substitute for it. Once you have a solid plan for action (literally), you can think about what to say, and, almost more importantly, what not to say.

Where to start

It is *always* worth the time and effort it takes to strengthen your rhythm. The first answer to every problem is always stronger rhythm. It may not be the only answer, but without it, everything else that you do will be standing on shaky ground.

When making changes to your rhythm, start with just one small piece of your day. Given how central rhythm is, you might be tempted to tackle the time of day with the biggest amount of stress and trouble. Do what you must, of course, but if you can, start with the transition that seems less challenging. Take small bites. Make a decision about one step that you can change – just one. Set yourself up for success by picking what seems easiest – although making changes is never really easy.

Sometimes it's best not to tackle a problem head on, but to come from another angle. In terms of transitions, if your biggest trouble spot is getting up in the morning, try putting your effort into going to bed. You may be surprised to find that working on the 'tails' side has a significant impact on the 'heads' side. If getting off to school is a hassle, attend to how your child returns. What does she come home to? What is her routine there? How could you adjust the emotional tone to better support her? Beginnings and endings are twins: you can't affect one without the other being influenced.

For more spontaneous people, routine may go against your grain but it matters to your children – a lot. Don't try to do it all. Try to find one regular routine that you can live with. If it is only once a week – pancakes on Sunday or pizza on Friday – that is a start. Your kids will be extra grateful for that one moment, that one solid period, in the long story of their week.

Paradoxically, when we make changes for the better, things can, at first, get worse. You may get full-blown meltdown and defiance. It is important to understand this dynamic, since the best-laid plans are often abandoned because people confuse that initial back-step as failure. Don't give up!

Chapter Six
Responsibilities: Doing chores together

Family life takes a lot of daily work. This is unlikely to be news to anyone who is reading this book. Expectations about *whose work this is* are a major part of the environment we create in our homes – the environment in which we bring up our children. Part of the structure of a household subtly shaping what each person can do and become is the division of work between family members. Ho Hum will be easier to put into practice if it is clear to everyone that we all pitch in. Children thrive in homes where family life is not regarded as something provided for children by parents, but where it is something the family all creates together. Of course parents lead and shoulder the lion's share of domestic tasks, especially when children are young, but Ho Hum is fostered where we assume that managing the household's daily needs is a shared effort in which every family member has a role.

Chores are closely connected to daily and weekly rhythm as discussed in the last chapter. Rhythm supports us in getting regular chores done, and chores become the cornerstones of your rhythm, providing moments when the family comes together to get a task done.

Must Chores be a Chore?

Sit at any youth sports event with parents, and you will hear the lamenting:

'I can't get my kids to do anything around the house.'

'I used to nag, nag, nag, and if I could get them to do anything at all, they did such a bad job that I stopped asking. It isn't worth it. Now I just do it myself.'

'My son said to me the other day: "Mom, you can't make me take the trash out. I am bigger than you."'

'My parents made me do so many chores that I couldn't get out of the house until Saturday afternoon, so I don't ask my kids to do much.'

The Buddhists say, 'Before enlightenment, chop wood and carry water; after enlightenment, chop wood and carry water.' Whether or not we are enlightened, the chores have to be done. The questions for parents are: Who does them and how? And, more important: why?

When we have to do something that we don't want to do, something dull and tedious, we describe it as being 'such a chore.' Chores have a bad reputation. Watch parents when they talk about them. Their shoulders sink. They seem tired and defeated. Or their jaws are tense. They are angry and frustrated. How children think of chores tends to depend on their parents. Kids with overly permissive parents tend to treat chores as something to weasel out of or at least something to be done with minimal effort. Kids with overly dominating parents tend to think of chores as a punishment or a contest of wills.

It doesn't have to be this way. Children can be ready, willing and able to do almost any chore. While I don't know of any kid who wakes up in the morning with a burning desire to scrub a toilet, it is possible that they will get the job done without nagging or pressure, that they will do the job well, and, on top of everything, that they will feel a real sense of satisfaction when they are done. When your children grow up and leave the house, it is possible that instead of feeling relieved that you no longer have to pick up after them, you are dismayed at how much you have to do again. You recognize just how much they contributed and how much you truly relied on them. In order to achieve this, we need to shift away from assuming that there will be resistance and away from thinking that we need to break through their resistance to doing chores.

We need to find a way for children to be motivated from within. Instead of being a battle of wills, doing chores, like other elements of our daily and weekly rhythm, can simply become a habit: something that is done regularly, with competence and efficiency.

Under Age Seven: Imitation and Invitation

Children under seven years are ripe for learning to do chores. You can teach older children to do chores, but they will learn them in a wholly different way. In a sense, for younger children, chores become a habit that they will absorb into their skin. It will become part of them, growing as they do, always a good fit, while older children will learn to put the habit on like a coat, something designed by someone else that they may be reluctant to wear at times.

Until children are seven, they learn by imitation: by using their bodies to do what they see others doing. It is learning on an unconscious level, and because of this, the learning is deeply internalized. There is no barrier. There is no stopping to consider what to take in and what to discard. All is absorbed.

This is such a powerful force that we adults are wise to take a good honest look at our own habits because we will see them – all of them – reflected in our children. It can be amusing when your little one sits down on the sofa to 'read' the paper and carefully arranges himself in exactly the same position in which you are sitting, crossing his legs just so, folding and smoothing the paper, even arranging his face into your frown of concentration. It is less flattering when you recognize your own voice as he complains to his stuffed animals, 'I have to do *everything* around here.'

To your young child, what you do is, by definition, important, interesting and worthwhile. Work with that. Expand on your child's natural inclinations to imitate by inviting your three or four year old to join you in your work.

Pull a chair up to the counter so he can help you stir, mash or chop. Let him sink his hands into warm, soapy dishwater. Stand beside him and wash a few things. Let him wash something that his little hands can grasp: a small plate or a mug. If he just wants to play with the suds, great. Later, he will associate that pleasure with doing dishes. After a meal, invite him to bring his empty bowl to the sink. When you go to wipe the table and chairs, hand him his own warm, damp cloth, saying simply, 'You may wipe your chair.' Hand him a scoop of dog food, 'You may put this in her bowl.' Hand him his own tiny jar of furniture wax ('You may...'), and he will apply it exactly as you do, at least for a moment, and then he may drop it all and run off. Let him wrestle with the vacuum cleaner, turning it on and off, dragging it around the carpet as he tries to master the balance of the pushing and the pulling. **At this stage, his help will not always be helpful, but you want to encourage his participation. You want him to feel that joining you in your work is a privilege, not a chore.**

Keep in mind that if you ask him whether he wants to put the cans of tomato sauce away in the cabinet, you encourage him to consider what he wants, setting yourself up for conflicts later on when he is required to do chores. So avoid orders that are camouflaged as requests, such as, 'Would you please put these away?' Leave it as an invitation to be accepted or not. At this age, instead of insisting, 'Here, put these on the shelf,' stick with: 'You may put these on the shelf.' If he does not take you up on the invitation, there is no harm done. There is no challenge to worry about. If there is no insistence, there is no resistance. Let his natural inclination to imitate lead him, but don't force it.

Do your work with care, deliberation, even joy. Let the siren song of your motion, your gestures, draw him in. Sing! Not only do work songs set a rhythm and cadence for chores, most of which involve repetitive motions, but they are uplifting and draw together all those involved with a sense of belonging and of common purpose (or choose any song – my husband favors R&B or punk rock, with some hilariously awful rewrites of the lyrics).

If you sing while you are working, it will keep you from filling the empty space with explanations. It is far better, at this stage, to allow your actions to speak for you. **If you explain what to do, you distract the child from the doing.** He will learn best if he can imitate, using his body purely and simply, without his conscious mind distracting him from his work.

If you are explaining something, your child will not so much be listening to what you say, but will be internalizing what you are doing: talking. This is why, so often, when parents later expect their children to do chores, instead of doing them, the children explain: usually all the reasons why they can't do them! They are, ironically, imitating their parents.

If we aren't going to explain things to children, what do we say? Think stories. Think pictures instead of concepts. Instead of 'Now it's time to put your toys away,' you could say: 'These toys are all worn out. Let's put them to bed, all snug and cozy, so they are ready to come out and play again later.' For an example of a complex conceptual instruction often given to young children, consider 'Be careful!' What does careful mean? It is a concept that we have to learn to apply to all sorts of situations – sometimes it means to slow down, sometimes it means to pay attention, and sometimes it means to not go near the edge or to stop. Try instead to be specific: create a picture with words. It is just like our high school English teachers tried to teach us: don't say it, show it. If you want your child to stir the pancake batter gently, instead of telling him to be careful, tell him that it is like stirring clouds: lift and turn the batter over.

When possible, child-sized tools can make doing chores more inviting for a child: not plastic imitations, the real thing only smaller. Giving a child plastic imitations of real tools makes a mockery of his ability to do real work. He cannot really turn a screw with a plastic screwdriver, and so he learns that his work won't produce actual results. With a tiny broom or a small spade, a child will not be overwhelmed by an implement that is too large and ungainly for him to handle, and he can see the real changes brought about by his efforts.

I once sent my four year old out with his spade to start digging a fire pit. We had marked the outline with stones, and I figured it would keep him busy for quite a while. About twenty minutes later, I went back out with my own shovel, expecting to help him get it done. I was too late. He had dug the whole thing. That night we built a roaring fire and roasted some marshmallows, and he savored the results of his industry.

Do not underestimate the ability of a small child to do real work. Invite him into your world of work. Be creative in looking for tasks where he can help. If it is too difficult or dangerous, look for a way to break it down and find some element in which he can participate. He might be too short to put away dishes, but he can stand on a chair and put the utensils in a drawer. He might not be able to sweep up all the dirt, but he can hold the dustpan for you. Folding shirts could be frustrating, but folding towels, making the corners 'kiss,' is do-able. He might not be able to hit the nails (he might!), but he can pass you nails as you need them. Let him feel the satisfaction that comes from hard, physical work. Invite him to carry heavy grocery bags, roll big rocks or logs in the yard and haul a full watering can or basket of laundry. Let his smaller size be an advantage: you can't squeeze behind the sofa to vacuum quite as well as he can. He can crawl under the bed to retrieve those socks with far more grace than you. Be a little clumsy. Let him 'help' you. Thank goodness he is there, otherwise, how would you possibly manage?

The best time to teach your children about using the hot stove and sharp knives is when they are young. This is the time when they will be the most careful, when your caution and care will have the most influence. They are just as physically capable of handling a knife at six as they will be when they are ten. If you wait until they are older, the risks are higher because an older child *thinks* he is more capable and is therefore less cautious. Teach them when they are young, when the habits of planting the point of the knife before slicing, of cutting away from the fingers, of turning the pot handle in, and so on, will be ingrained deeply into their physical memory. You don't have to give them a cleaver or a hatchet but, with supervision, a six year old should be able to handle using a paring knife and stirring a pot on a hot stove.

While children under seven are not ready to be held accountable for doing regular household chores (taking out the trash, doing dishes, hauling wood and such), they should be encouraged as early as possible to clean up after themselves and to take part in their basic self-care. This means picking up toys as well as self-care tasks such as getting dressed, brushing teeth and hair, making their beds, hanging up their bath towels, clearing their plates from the table, and putting dirty clothes in the laundry hamper. **Don't leave them alone to clear up after themselves, but once they can do it, they really should most of the time. This is the 'doing with' stage.** They are still little. They will need you there at the sink while they brush their teeth. They will need you there turning down the other side of the bed. They will need you there encouraging them to 'make the basket' with their dirty socks.

Loving gestures of warmth and generosity, such as combing a child's hair, will be long remembered and cherished. Just watch that, in your bounding love for him, you don't do everything for him. If he is tired or if a shirt has especially difficult buttons, by all means help him, but let him do as much as he is able. If you continue to do these tasks for the child after he is able to do them for himself, you imply that it is your job, one that he might help with occasionally when he feels like it, but not one that he is responsible for. Not only is he robbed of the satisfaction of knowing that he can, in fact, take care of these things, he will always be looking for someone else to do it.

Keep your eyes out for signs that he wants to try on his own. Sometimes we continue to help because we want something done 'right.' We want the shoes on the right feet, the sheets tucked just so, the shirt facing the front. Be willing to accept some awkwardness in his attempts. This is the time to celebrate effort, not results.

As for cleaning up toys, remember that this is still a time when the child's strongest impulse is to imitate. It is a time of 'doing with.' If you send him off to do it on his own, you invite a struggle. You must be willing to do it alongside him with warmth and enthusiasm. This requires discipline on your part because you will have to be consistent. Think this one through. Be realistic about what you are going to expect.

If you want your child to learn to pick up after he is done, you will have to help him do that – every time. That means noticing when he is done, stopping whatever you are doing, and enlisting him in the task. (Using imaginative language is very helpful here, creating a story or image to make it more fun and lighten the burden.) It may also work for you to have a set time when things are picked up: after lunch, before dinner, whatever works for you. But you are the key. In order to develop a habit, he must do the same thing over and over. That means you must do it, too, so know your own limitations and set your child and yourself up for success.

Bite off what you can chew. Pick one thing to work on at a time and build from there. It doesn't have to happen all at once. It is consistency you are aiming for, even in one very small area. That is where the habit will root itself, and you can add to it as you are able.

Something to consider: if your child has a hard time putting away toys, he may have too many of them. We are so accustomed to thinking that more of a good thing is better. Not always.

Harness the power of rhythm. Doing chores at regular times of the day or week supports your child's developing habits. Take some time to consider when in your day and your week it makes the most sense to get chores done. For most people, getting up in the morning, mealtimes and bedtime are the areas where they tend to be the most consistent. Attach your chores to the points in the day with the strongest rhythm. In this way, the habit of doing those tasks can ride on the coattails of the settled, motivated rhythm of, say, your meals. You will find that later, when you assign chores to your children, this connection to your regular daily and weekly pattern will make the process far easier.

Why Bother? Why chores are so important

If teaching your children to do chores sounds time-consuming to you, you are right. It is. All tasks take longer at this stage if you meaningfully include your children. You might wonder if it is worth teaching your child to do chores at all. It can be easier to do them ourselves. Some people hire someone to do them if they can afford it. What is there to lose? A lot, actually. **Your investment of time right now will reap exponential rewards later, for you and your child.**

Learning to do chores at an early age is essential to the development of a healthy will. This is entirely different from willfulness, where children are primarily concerned with resistance or getting their own way. A child with a healthy will expects that the needs of the day, including his, are the top priority, and he takes comfort in the certainty of this. Not only does he sense the rightness of this, but he is willing to put his abilities toward the task. The child has a sense of inevitability, of being buoyed along by the day's events guided by you, the parent.

Your gentle guidance, day after day, builds a solid foundation upon which your child will develop his character. The base of that foundation is made of gratitude. If we look to cultivate any one quality in our young children, gratitude would be the place to start. Gratitude is the seed out of which love grows and flourishes – love for you and others close to your child, as well as those with whom he has only incidental contact: the bagger at the grocery store, the man who collects the trash, and the woman who drives the bus. Gratitude is the seed of love for all the living and inanimate beings that share his world: the sun and sky, the trees and rocks and birds. It is also the ground for self-esteem – for loving himself.

How is it that something as simple and mundane as picking up one's towel or clearing one's dishes can give rise to gratitude? It is because we must understand that we have been given gifts before we can feel grateful for them. It is not so much living in the cleanliness or orderliness that leads to gratitude as it is the realization of how much effort goes into the work of the day. It is having a sense of the hands that folded the pile of clean laundry waiting to be put away, that chopped and grated and rolled to create that plate of steaming enchiladas. Gratitude comes from a feeling of being welcomed into the greater current of life.

A child who does not pick up after himself, who does not learn to contribute and share in the daily work of his household, will have a fundamentally different view of the world than the child who is taught that he has a part to play, that he is relied upon as well as cherished. The first child will feel that the world exists to serve him, that he is somehow separate and above those around him. He will have learned that all of those daily tasks belong to someone else (us), and when we expect him to take on some of those tasks, he will resent it, feeling that we are somehow slacking on our job and are trying to get him to fill the void. This is not conducive to feeling grateful.

The second child will have a much stronger sense of the interdependence among the people of his world, and he will feel that he belongs in that vast web. If we draw the young child warmly and with companionship into the world of chores, he will understand that ultimately we all carry responsibility, and he will be willing, even eager, to shoulder his part. As he matures, as he finds his place in the world and discerns his calling in life, this healthy will enables him to act, taking up that life's work.

Age Seven to Fourteen: Assigned chores

Once children reach the age of seven, they are ready for assigned chores, but this is not the time to hand your child a list and walk away. He will need a gradual shift from being invited to join in a task to being expected to start it and complete it on his own. If you have a rhythm established, he will have internalized the basic pattern of the day, and that is a great place to start. If you don't have a rhythm established, attend to that first and give yourself plenty of time to do that. Hurrying is antithetical to rhythm, so allow yourself a bit of a grace period to put your house in order. I am thinking in terms of months or a year, not days or weeks. Seriously, the rhythm is that important.

With rhythm established, the only change you need to make is a gradual handing over of tasks. What gets done and when it gets done remains the same. The goal now is to divide up the tasks among all the people of the household, with your child gradually handling more as he grows. Think of this stage as a time when each member of the household attends to individual parts of a task with the task being done all together as a group. **It is still a time of 'doing with,' but instead of doing the same task together, everyone works together on separate tasks.**

Dividing Up the Work: One Example

By way of example, I will describe how our family divided up the group chores when our children were aged seven to fourteen. Ours is not the only way, just one way.

DAILY

Cleaning up after meals: Everyone brought their own plates to the sink. For breakfast and lunch, I filled the sink with warm, soapy water and everyone washed their own personal dishes and put them in the dish rack, which I later emptied. I usually took care of pots and pans. For dinner, we all cleared the table, and then one washed all the dishes and pots (my husband or I to start, but everyone cycled through), one dried, one put away dishes and one put away leftovers and wiped the table. The dog cleaned up the floor.

Feeding/caring for animals: My son fed the dog, and my daughter took care of the chickens. I took care of the horses, with help from my daughter. We did these chores right before or after breakfast, so that it was easy to remember them.

Meal preparation: Unless I cooked something, Sunday pancakes for breakfast or a hot lunch, my children prepared their own breakfast and lunch and then we all sat down together. That included wiping up the counter after they were done and putting ingredients away. I cooked dinner, with occasional help from either child when they were there: chopping, mixing, setting the table. My daughter liked to help mostly with baking. My son favored making sauces (and wow! Sometimes he got really 'creative' with the spices). I did the grocery shopping, but they would help unload the car and the bags. My husband usually emptied the compost in the winter, and I did it in the summer. Now that I think of it, I am not exactly sure how he got stuck with that one!

WEEKLY

Trash/recycling: We rotated this one. Most often it was my son who did it, since feeding the dog was a two-second job and the chickens required far more time.

Cleaning the house: Each child was responsible for keeping his or her room reasonably clean. They had relatively few playthings, and they generally picked up after themselves, so when it was time to clean the house, we didn't have to spend much time straightening up before getting down to the actual cleaning.

Our children started with cleaning bathroom sinks and counters (while my husband and I cleaned something else). Using a spray bottle gives that job some semblance of fun. Toilets were added in relatively quickly. No one should be afraid of a toilet. The kitchen was cleaned after dinner along with dishes. Dusting seems easy but takes a lot of attention to detail, and it is the job most hated by my kids. They each had to do a stint, just to know how to do it (a stint being about three months without any major complaining). We had two floors, so they started out vacuuming just one.

I helped them do all of these at the start until they had the hang of it, and then they usually told me that they didn't need me there, and I would go off to finish up my part. We cleaned the house on Saturday morning, when all of us were home. It never took us more than an hour. I personally detest vacuuming and will be devastated when my son leaves the house, since, aside from being delightful, he has taken that job for years. Our policy is that you don't have to do a job you can't stand – but only after you have successfully and cheerfully done it for a while.

I like to get the house clean all at once and then steadfastly refuse to clean during the week unless someone throws up or a potato explodes in the oven. For some, splitting up the cleaning chores over the week is more manageable, with the bathrooms being done one day, the vacuuming another and so on. (And anyone with an infant: remember that getting a load of laundry done and showering in one day is a superhuman effort worthy of applause.)

There are some folks whose temperament just will never sit well with a plan at all. That is OK. For you, a cleaning fire drill can be very effective (and can be a welcome change even for those who like a routine). A cleaning fire drill is a random, short burst of cleaning. Announced with something loud and dramatic (banging on a pot with a spoon works), the fire drill involves fifteen minutes of speedy cleaning with all hands on deck. It is a race against time to get as much done before the alarm sounds again. You will be surprised at how much you can accomplish in such little time – proof that most of the time we associate with cleaning is really procrastination.

Laundry: Everyone put his/her laundry in the hamper, and I washed it on Mondays and Fridays. Once we were past the infant stage when laundry was a daily event, having this twice-weekly rhythm helped me to not feel consumed by laundry. There was a day to do it, and the rest of the time I would sail past the pile: later for you. In the warmer months, I would hang it out on the line, and this was one of my favorite times. We were lucky to live in a beautiful place, and spending a few moments out at the laundry line, watching cranes dance in the field beyond the fence and listening to the comforting sound of the horses grinding grass in their teeth was like a meditation for me, so I never shared that job, and no one ever complained.

I folded the laundry and everyone took their pile and put it away. When my daughter was about ten or twelve (how is it that I can't keep track of that stuff?), I could no longer distinguish her socks from mine, so she started doing her own. My son began doing his when he was fourteen, when he and my husband wore the same size boxers. (His entry into the laundry world was imminent anyway, but he precipitated it by complaining quite peevishly when I mistakenly washed his red soccer jersey with his white soccer socks, which came out pink.) But he took being given the job as a sign of his greater maturity, as it truly was. He now goes cheerfully thumping down the stairs with his loads, and I have to fill out my husband's and my bundle with towels to make a full load.

SEASONAL

Winter: In the winter, there was firewood to be split, stacked and hauled inside as well as snow to be shoveled. My son had a love for wood and learned how to use an axe to split it somewhere around the age of ten. He wasn't required to do the wood chores, but he liked to. Otherwise, my husband and I did it. I don't recall my daughter being involved too much.

Spring and Fall: In the spring and again in the fall, the garden was the big push. Both children helped out in various ways, but neither was required to do so.

Summer: In the summer the lawn needed mowing, and the kids took that over when they were about ten or twelve, each mowing half. Before that, mowing was my job (my husband did the irrigating, fence mending, harrowing, and more). Sometimes I used to do the mowing when I was frazzled and couldn't stand my kids. They would come out and try to get my attention, and I would just smile and wave and point to my ears: 'Sorry, I can't hear you!' The lawn got mowed, and I always felt better afterward and could respond with more patience.

Sharing the Load

You can divide up your chores however you want, but I want to draw your attention to some important details. My husband and I had an informal division of labor. As it turned out, it was fairly traditional, but it wasn't intentionally so. We just stuck to our strengths, but you will notice that with the cleaning up, the daily dishes and the weekly housecleaning, my husband was there, sharing in the work (and contributing colorful commentary; he does talk for a living). I am fairly certain that enlisting Dad's participation in cleaning is the single most motivating element for children. **Regardless of the make-up of your family, the key here is that when group chores are tackled, it**

CHAPTER SIX: RESPONSIBILITIES

is essential that everyone do them. There is no one sitting out. This sends an unmistakable message that cleaning up is everyone's job. They are not just helping Mom with 'her' job. No matter who cooked, we all cleaned up after dinner.

We very consciously scheduled our housecleaning for a time when we were all home. Interestingly, after many years of all four of us cleaning the house together, my children and I came to a consensus that, since we three were home more, and we no longer wanted to use up our weekend time with cleaning, we would take care of housecleaning earlier in the day during the week, when my husband was at work. While this meant more work for each of us, we all felt it was a worthwhile trade. He still helped with the dishes after dinner.

Another note about Dad: If you are tempted to put this book down right now and march into the living room to tell your husband, 'It's all your fault that the kids don't do chores! Now you get to do the laundry,' resist that temptation. Enlist his help, don't demand it. Let him know how important his contribution is. If it is a stretch for him to participate for whatever reason, see if you can find just one short moment in the day when you all can accomplish a chore together. It could be all of you bringing in the groceries or clearing the table after dinner. Make a point of playing up the doing-it-together aspect. It is the fact that the work is shared that matters, not the amount that is accomplished.

How Much Is Enough?

If you have children under seven and you are overwhelmed by chores, you are just normal. Young children, while being delightful beyond words, can also be a test of our endurance. Raising children is not for the faint of heart. The laundry alone can make one weep. Rhythm helps, but the truth is that there is simply a lot of work to be done. Keep your eye on the long-term goals: help is on the way. If you have children over seven and you are overwhelmed by chores, your children need to be doing more. When in doubt, more chores are better than less.

Where is the balance? I do know some folks whose parents seemed to use chores as a method of domination. They were given endless chores, which were obviously designed as busywork. The red flag in these situations was that the children were working and the parents weren't. Your guide, at this stage, is to look around during chore time and see who is not participating. Whatever chores you have designated as group chores (and I would suggest that housecleaning and meal clean-up be the baseline) should be done by everyone at the same time. Adjust for age and ability by giving a smaller, easier part of the task to the younger children, but anyone over seven should be involved.

What about balancing chores with extra-curricular activities? These days, it is so easy – too easy – for children's days to be so completely chock-full of lessons, sports activities, clubs and more, that there is no time for them to do chores. Families make huge sacrifices in their finances and time in order to make these activities possible. Because this is so, in order to maintain that healthy will and not foster selfishness, it is doubly important that your children regularly attend to their chores. No one should be so special that they need not take out the trash.

Standards: What is Reasonable?

What sorts of standards are reasonable? Washing dishes, taking out the trash, mopping a floor – all of these are skills that must be taught, and they take time to learn, just like any other skill. That means that you need to help your child practice until he has mastered it. Be there, showing him how, encouraging him, letting him try it out. Accept awkward attempts at first, as long as he is making an effort. He will let you know when he has got it. Once he has mastered it, expect a reasonable job.

Since you are all working together, it is easy enough to poke your head into the bathroom or wherever and check on progress. If it is really substandard, you can just let your child know, in a matter-of-fact way, that it is not yet acceptable. Treat it as an oversight on his part, whether it is deliberate or not. It doesn't matter, since he must do it reasonably well, regardless. Focus on the job, not the attitude.

Does he need help or is he just having a bad attitude? Sometimes what we think is a bad attitude is a disguise for feeling inadequate. Only you can determine whether he is over his head and needs a smaller task or more coaching, or if he is simply feigning incompetence in hopes of getting out of doing the job altogether. By using Ho Hum – gentle but firm expectation that he complete the task and a kind willingness to offer the guidance necessary to help him do that – he will find that resistance, including a bad attitude, just makes the inevitable take longer.

Sometimes a child will try outright refusal. Well, let's be real: they all try it. Who wouldn't? **Ho Hum is the key, as always. The challenge is that you can't actually *make* anyone do anything. But it is possible to not allow them to do anything else until the job is done.** A simple, 'You may _____ (fill in the blank: have lunch, play outside) as soon as you are done,' is all that is called for. No further explanations, no bargains, no exhortations about attitudes. Ho Hum. That is just the way it is. His resistance is not a moral failing. It is just a mistake, an attempt to see what will happen.

It is your job to let him know what will happen: nothing, until the job is done. Whining, temper tantrums, any sort of reaction, if handled with Ho Hum, will simply waste the child's time (and yours, but you don't want to let them know that) but will not buy him any sort of reprieve from doing the job and doing it right. When the drama is over, the chore is still waiting, and 'as soon as' it is done, he is free to carry on. The only exception to that rule would be for bedtime or school. But the chore would be waiting first thing in the morning or right after school, and he could wait in his room until he is ready to do it.

Paying Children to Do Chores

Paying your children to do chores or giving them allowance and tying it to chores, which is just another version of paying them to do it, is a bad idea. The whole point of chores, aside from being training in necessary life skills, is to develop a healthy will, a will to share the burden and contribute to the family life as a whole. If a child only does a chore if he is paid, his motivation becomes a selfish one, exactly the opposite of the primary reason for teaching him to do chores in the first place. It implies that it is someone else's job, only worth his while if he is given enough money for it. Resist the temptation. What may seem like a great way to enlist his cooperation now will likely backfire later. Once you pay your child for a job, you set yourself up for more resistance. Ho Hum is much more effective in the long term, and it is cheaper, too.

What If I Started Late?

What if you missed the window, before age seven, to initiate doing chores using the power of imitation? All is not lost. Your job will be harder, it is true, but it can be done. Your child will most likely resist the introduction of assigned chores with more insistence and tenacity than a child who learned early that doing them is just part of life. Your child has learned that doing chores is *not* part of life, and it will take time to undo that. Be prepared to get lots of practice using Ho Hum.

Without your young child's natural inclination to imitate, he will necessarily need more direct guidance and explanation – and lots of encouragement. Make sure that the chores are being done as a group, use Ho Hum to avoid a contest of wills, and in this case, Dad's participation is crucial. I would say that his participation alone can make or break it.

Chores and Teenagers

Once your children reach adolescence, they will have mastered all of the regular household chores and will hopefully have a fairly well established habit of doing them, supported by the momentum of the whole family working together. **This is the time to let them choose when to do their assigned chores, to allow them more flexibility and control.** As long as they are responsible, they can have the freedom, within agreed upon limits, to do the task when it fits their schedule.

You will likely have to contract and expand this freedom in response to how well your teen handles it. Use Ho Hum. If he fails, the consequence is that he must go back to doing his chores with the group. He can try again in a few weeks. A chore list is appropriate now, but remember that it is only as effective as you are in following through.

At this point, if your child has developed a healthy will, he may not always look forward to his chores – few do – but he will have accepted them in his world and will feel a strong sense of belonging, a sense that he has an important role and is relied upon. He will welcome the increased responsibility as a sign of, and acknowledgment of, his greater maturity.

Where to Start

If your children have not been involved with chores and are over seven years old, start out with the 'doing with' approach. Pick one chore – cleaning up dinner, for example – and divide the job into as many parts as you have people over seven, then work together to get it done. It is more important to do one chore together than it is to do anything else. This includes self-care. If they haven't cleaned their room with you helping to start with, don't expect them to do it on their own. They must experience the lifting tide of working together. In this case, I would allow grumpiness as long as it didn't spill over into disrespectful words.

Chapter Seven
Creating an Environment for Play:
Sharing and generosity

The last chapter looked at how our expectations about work inside our families can have a powerful impact. This chapter looks at our expectations about play, and how to avoid hampering our children's happy and productive play even as we are trying to foster it.

It's often said that play is children's work: they learn and grow through play. Play is how they express their responses to the world, and where they unconsciously seek solutions to their problems, big and small. Setting up a social and physical environment in which children can settle into their own play is at the core of parenting. It is of great benefit to your children, and thus also to you, as having freedom to play will reduce your child's frustration, and assist in developing her social self and her ability to negotiate with others – including, of course, you.

We can create an environment that fosters play by asking careful questions about the toys we provide, and about what positive negotiation with others actually looks like. Many of our most influential assumptions about play involve sharing.

What Happens When we Force Children to 'Share'?

Pete is sitting in the sand surrounded by a few buckets, shovels and plastic lizards. He is playing with a car, zooming it over obstacles and around hairpin turns, each change in speed or direction accompanied by appropriate sound effects and play-by-play analysis. Bobby, drawn to what is obviously fun and absorbing, comes over and tries to obtain the car for himself. Depending on his temperament, Bobby will try the direct grab, a polite request to share (rare, but it does happen) or something in between. Pete, not nearly done with this particular racing event, refuses, using one of many methods of doing so, ranging from ignoring Bobby to bopping him on the head with the car.

At this point, Bobby goes for back-up: the responsible adult. Just sitting and crying loudly is effective, but once a child is fairly verbal, the time-honored technique is some version of 'Mo-om, he won't share.' Mom, seeing that Bobby wants the toy car and that Pete is not forthcoming, says, 'OK, Pete, you have to share. Two more minutes to play with the car and then give Bobby a turn.'

How many times have you witnessed a variation of the above? We all want our kids to share. No one wants their child to be greedy. Generosity is the foundation of friendship, and when our kids don't share, we imagine them lonely and isolated, surrounded by the toys they hogged, which are poor substitutions for companionship. And so we make them share.

Let's take a step back and look at this scenario again. What exactly are we teaching our children when we make them share? And will these lessons help them to become generous? Let's be honest. Pete would be an unusual child if, after his two minutes are up and Bobby is now getting a turn with the car, he were to think to himself, 'Boy, Bobby sure is enjoying that car. Next time he wants it, I will hand it right over. This sharing is great!'

First, can I suggest that sharing is a fairly advanced concept and that few adults agree on what constitutes appropriate sharing. Witness our current political strife. How would you feel if your neighbor came over and asked to use your lawnmower while you were mowing your lawn, and you were told that you had two more minutes and then had to give it over? Think of all the times a neighbor has come over to borrow a shovel, a ladder, an egg. Depending on the neighbor, you might be comfortable with that, but what about your bicycle, your car or some of your bank account? Where is the line?

Pete may, in fact, learn that he has to share when told to do so, but that will not often plant the seed of generosity in his heart. More likely, he will be nursing a budding resentment. Play is not just any old activity for children. It is a planet, a world apart. Lost in his own world of car racing, Pete is arbitrarily jerked out of it because Bobby wants the car.

We always seem to focus on and exert pressure on the child who has the toy, but we rarely consider the longer-term needs of the child who wants the toy. There are better ways to encourage Pete to include Bobby, but, more importantly, what lessons does Bobby learn when we force Pete to share with him? Why did Bobby need to have the car that Pete was playing with? Was that the only toy available? Why is Bobby's desire more important than Pete's?

Forcing Pete to share is very unlikely to foster his internal motivation to share in the future. What's more, it is going to reinforce two lessons for Bobby that we might want to avoid: 'I want, therefore I must have,' and 'Things are more important than people.' Neither of these invites empathy, which is the foundation for generosity.

Sometimes parents will approach this situation by trying to teach the boys to communicate, suggesting that Bobby ask nicely for the car, or the adult will model the asking: 'Pete, would you please share the car?' But this is not a genuine request, since it is very unlikely Pete would be allowed to say no. If Pete does hand over the car, everyone sighs in relief, feeling that cooperation has been furthered. But has it? In order for there to be cooperation, there must be some element of mutual understanding, of choice. Pete had no choice here. He has just been pressured into an action. In this situation, cooperation means doing what the adult wants, and in this case, clearly the adult prefers that Bobby have the car. **Forced sharing has more to do with power than generosity.**

Being forced to share and to give up his own play is not going to endear Bobby to Pete, and it will likely mean that next time Pete has the car, he will be less able to enjoy playing with it. He will either devote significant time and attention to staking his claim: hoarding, going further away from where other kids are playing or acting aggressively. Alternatively, he will give up and be prepared to lose it at any moment, which prevents him from creating and being absorbed in his imaginative world. Any potential for developing a sense of warmth and connection between the two boys is lost. Both have learned that sharing is a contest with winners and losers.

Focus on Play, Not Sharing

We would consider it very bad manners if someone were to walk through a row of empty chairs and ask another person to give up her seat. It is appropriate to choose from the available chairs. And it is appropriate for children to do the same with playthings.

Try focusing on Bobby, 'the wanter.' Your task is to change his focus to a toy that is free. A simple statement from you is all that is called for: 'You may play with that when Pete is done. Let's see, here is another car.' Or you can guide Pete to speak for himself: 'Yes, you can have it when I am done.'

This is a simple yet significant shift, but simple doesn't mean easy. At first, it may not go smoothly. We tend to want to handle sharing conflicts in a way that causes the least amount of tears and fussing, but, unfortunately, this desire can lead us to the quick fix of forced sharing, which has negative long-term consequences.

Children who are accustomed to getting what they want will put up resistance if they are expected to wait or to find something else. This is the time to apply the principles of Ho Hum. Be firm, kind and patient. Understand that the child may well test you to see if you really mean it, to see if you can be swayed into going back to forcing sharing. But when a child has exhausted all avenues of convincing you to change your mind and you continue to remain pleasant and unmoved, he will accept the reality of the situation and settle down to play. There is light at the end of the tunnel. If you are consistent in not forcing sharing and in redirecting the 'wanter' to what is available *and* you do so with Ho Hum, the conflicts, and hence the drama, will diminish significantly.

When first introduced to the idea that sharing shouldn't be forced, many parents have their own resistance to the idea. They expect that Pete will prolong his use of the car, knowing that it will upset Bobby. This may happen at first, particularly if it causes a lot of drama. Without the drama, Pete will play with the car as long as his interest in it holds but no longer. In fact, if all the other children are busy playing with other things, he will enjoy his car more and will feel more relaxed and secure, which lays the foundation for him eventually sharing out of his own free will.

As far as Bobby is concerned, he will ultimately also feel more relaxed and secure if his playing is not dependent on his ability to obtain a toy from someone else, if he learns to focus on *playing* instead of *having*. The petty manipulations that are so prevalent in situations involving forced sharing will vanish fairly quickly if there is no drama to feed them.

You can let sharing be something that comes from your children freely when they are ready and able. Beware of reinforcing for Bobby that the only way to play and have fun is to possess one particular toy. If you put all your efforts into working out for the boys how to share that one toy, you affirm the toy's central importance. Chances are good that there are plenty of other toys to play with, and chances are even better that if Pete were not playing with that car, it might not have such a strong draw for Bobby.

Encourage your child to look for what is available. Very young children can often be distracted away from an 'attractive nuisance' – i.e.: the toy someone else is playing with, but as they get older, this is harder to do. When children are a bit older, they have learned what the rest of the world knows, which is that the best indicator of something's worth is that someone else has it. In that case, Bobby doesn't want just any car; he wants Pete's car. Either way, your task is to guide Bobby to a free toy and state simply, 'You may play with the other car when it is available.'

Remember that going for what someone else is using is not necessarily greed. It can just be that our attention naturally gravitates toward what someone else has or is doing. My friend and I once took our three year olds to an apple orchard. For an hour or so, we were the only people there, the twenty acres of trees ours for the literal picking. We wandered from tree to tree, looking for apples that had not been damaged by the recent hail, and stopped at a promising one. As my friend and I filled our bags and our little ones busied themselves in the grass, a car slowly drove up the dirt road and rolled to a stop just at the row where we were. A handful of people clambered out of the car and began walking down the row toward us. My friend and I joked about how, out of all the rows available, they had to choose the one where we were. Much to our surprise and amusement, the group continued down our row until they reached us and began picking from the very same tree!

Gravitating towards others and relying on someone else's judgment (in this case, our choice of trees) is simply human. If we can understand this basic tendency while we guide children to see the alternatives around them, we can do it without the added burden of judging them or labeling them. Learning to see and value what is around us can take some imagination and confidence. And that can take time. Be willing to help children with this until they can do it themselves.

Parents are sometimes advised to ask their child to pick out and set aside certain toys that are just too difficult to share, but this plants an image in the child's mind that some things are too special to share. It leads her to consider whether she wants to share or not, and it is better to not invite her to think along those lines. However, the idea behind the suggestion is sound: you want to make it easier for the children to play, and if you know your child will fall apart if someone picks up her special doll when she is not playing with it, better to leave the doll at home. But I would suggest not calling attention to this. Just do it. Generally, you know what is too special for your child to share, and you can just put it away when kids come over, or not bring it to the park.

What about taking turns? That is a bit of a grey area. Watch out for the slippery slope here. Taking turns may be appropriate for things like sliding down a slide or going across monkey bars. Expecting kids to take turns with a smaller object, one of those big plastic cars that they can ride in, for example, is getting awfully close to forcing sharing: 'Two minutes and then hand it over.' If there is one large item, a swing for example, it can be useful to have a timer and establish at the beginning that those who want to use it will take turns. Avoid encouraging any sort of jockeying for power or attention by not getting drawn into conflicts over turns.

Setting the Stage for Playing: Toys

When you are at home or have some control over children's surroundings, it is wise to structure the environment so that it can support their play. When we ask ourselves how best to encourage play, we tend to think that the answer lies directly with the children, but there are two other key elements that are often overlooked: the toys and you, the adult.

Let's start first with the toys. If ever a scapegoat is needed, instead of condemning a particularly aggressive or whiney child as the one causing all the trouble, blame the toys. Seriously. The stump that could be a castle, a stove, a dueling partner or a driver's seat has been replaced with a big plastic kitchen, complete with sink, cabinets and oven that can be used as... a sink, cabinets and oven. The square of bright fabric that could be used as a wedding veil, magic carpet, cape or tent has been replaced by a Batman costume that can be used as – you guessed it – a Batman costume. The sticks that could be swords, magic wands or goal posts, which could be fashioned into forts, bridges or doll beds, have been replaced with very realistic, usually plastic toys whose purpose is immediately obvious and is therefore fixed. Gone are the open-ended objects that could be anything or everything with only a bit of imagination.

While this is a detriment to child's play in many ways, it is very specifically a detriment to children learning to play primarily with each other instead of each other's toys. Think about it: **open-ended toys expand the supply of available toys exponentially. Any one object can be a thousand toys.**

A big plastic castle for every child would be expensive as well as unwise, but a big assortment of cardboard boxes? The possibilities are endless, limited only by the children's imaginations, which, given the opportunity, will prove boundless. Pete has a boat (a piece of bark) to float in a puddle and Bobby wants it? How about another piece of bark? Now they can both float their boats. The key is that these objects require an imaginative investment by the child, enough to turn the pillow into a doll bed or the laundry basket into a bucking bronco. You just don't see children angling for possession of these objects in the same way that they do realistic toys. Realistic toys limit children, making them more aware of and dependent on the toy, on what they have. Open-ended toys provide myriad options, freeing the children from being tied down to a single possibility dictated by a thing.

When children are immersed in the imaginative aspect of play, this shifts their attention away from the toys. Toys become a means to an end, instead of being the end. The objective is no longer to compete with Pete to win his car but to construct the entire racetrack, parking garage, and concession stand. There is so much to consider: how many lanes? Will they use a flag or gun to start the race? Maybe it turns out that horses race here as well, and that opens up a whole other world to construct. Pete is busy with his car? That is just fine. Bobby is busy with his own world. Maybe Pete will join him, maybe not, but both boys are busy playing.

Setting the Stage for Playing: Your Purposeful Activity

The second element to consider when setting the stage for play is what you (and any other adults present) are doing while the children are playing. Does it matter? It turns out: yes, tremendously. Even while they may seem to be totally engrossed, children are keenly aware of what the adults around them are doing.

Have you ever tried to sneak a treat while your kids were busy playing, only to have them right there, 'What'cha got, Mom?' Have you ever tried to move to the next bench when you are at the playground, and your toddler, who was happily packing sand into a bucket, bursts into tears and runs to you, clinging to your knees, no longer able to bear the ten foot distance between you? How about a phone call: when you pick up the phone, do your children immediately get into a fight?

What you are doing, where your attention is focused, matters. Does your child play better when you are on the phone or when you are at the sink doing dishes? At the sink, you are engaged in a useful activity, your hands are busy, your body is relaxed but in motion. Your attention is on what you are doing, but not entirely so. You are able to keep a quiet, barely discernible connection humming between you and your child. When the phone rings, that subtle bond is broken, your attention is pulled entirely away, your purposeful motion is replaced by the staccato of conversation, and the holding power of the rhythm within the activity is cut: hence the fight or the fuss.

Our presence can be part of the supportive environment in which the child plays. Think of what you are doing as the theme underlying a piece of music. The children literally will feel the pulse of that and take their cues from it. The children's play is borne on that current. They are swept along by it, involved in creating their own scenarios, their own little melodies. They are too engrossed – too busy actually – to be diverted by the discordant notes of competition for toys.

The basic ingredient for creating that current, that theme, is for

you to be engaged in some kind of purposeful activity while the children play. So you don't have to do dishes, but that is about the level of activity that you are aiming for: something that involves your hands and is relatively quiet, and that draws your eyes away from the children without claiming all of your attention or awareness.

Knitting, mending, weeding, chopping vegetables, hanging or folding laundry: chores essentially. Working on a computer? Nope. It is too engrossing, and there is not enough body engagement. It is the same with the phone. Sitting with other moms and conversing won't cut it either, unless possibly if you all have some sort of handwork project to do. My children would say that since I wave my hands around so much when I talk that it might qualify for me, but no. Purposeful activity means an activity that the *children* can discern as purposeful. Also, like the phone, conversation alone tends to draw us in so completely that we lose our awareness. We sever the thread.

The benefit of your purposeful activity is twofold: it keeps you from either hovering or abandoning. Hovering too closely over the children, being ready to jump in at the first sign of trouble, stifles children and makes them self-conscious. It encourages them to be hypersensitive to any sign of conflict, it invites the children to draw you into conflicts, and it is simply distracting, keeping them from immersing themselves in their play.

The opposite of hovering is leaving the children to their own devices so that they must come up with their own solutions if conflicts arise. There are some contexts in which this can work, but too often this leaves the children vulnerable to the same sort of power dynamics that occur when sharing is forced, where one child wins and another loses.

Your engagement in your own activity sets the tone for the children to attend to their own activity. Setting the tone: we use this phrase without understanding what it means, and so we don't harness it as we might. When you put yourself in motion, it is like call and response. Without being conscious of it, the children will sense your rhythm, your intention: the tone. They will hear the underlying beat, and they will respond with something similar. Their innate drive to imitate will take hold of them and propel them forward. It reassures them and frees them at the same time. This is why what you choose to do has such an impact.

Does this mean that you can never sit down and pay the bills or talk with a friend or just relax? No. You don't always have to be so consciously engaged. But for the times when you are unsure of how your child will respond – situations involving new kids, new places or new activities, or times when anyone is tired or stressed – your engagement in purposeful activity while the children play can be a lifesaver.

Fostering Generosity

Generosity, the unselfish giving or sharing of what one has, is born out of a feeling of security within oneself and a feeling of empathy for another. All children have the potential to act generously. It is not something that we have to put in but is more something that needs caretaking so that it can flourish on its own. By not forcing sharing, you will protect your child from associating the act of giving with a feeling of resentment or powerlessness. This opens the door to feelings of companionship, which is the soil out of which empathy will grow.

When giving grows out of a sense of warmth and connection, when it is not imposed from the outside but encouraged to develop from within, the one doing the giving learns the truth about generosity: that it offers the giver as much pleasure or even more, than the recipient.

If generosity is treated as a privilege, not an obligation, other important lessons can also be learned. One concerns boundaries: we want our children to learn to give that which is healthy and right for them, but no more. We want them to be able to resist coercion and negative influence. Learning to give in response to their own impulse reinforces a healthy set of boundaries. Second, it teaches them that a gift comes from the heart and is not a bargaining chip. A true gift has no strings attached, no expectation of reciprocity. If there is an exchange, the child will be delighted and grateful, but she will not be resentful if there is not. This is fundamental to true generosity.

Where to Start

Since small children learn primarily by imitating those around them, we would do well to model generosity and sharing ourselves. Grandiose gestures may be beyond their ability to absorb or copy, but small gestures sprinkled about will be noticed. Food is often the first gift and the easiest: offering snacks to friends, putting food out for birds, feeding a pet, bringing a meal to an older neighbor. Offering our time in the service of another is especially significant. As our children grow, our examples will not be lost on them. Keep up the good work!

To support your children's play, perhaps try adding a few open-ended toys to their environment. When transitioning from realistic toys to ones that require (and nourish) imagination, I find that bigger is better. For an outdoor setting, see if you can find some large stumps, long sticks, boards or planks, and big stones. For an indoor setting, my personal favorite is a giant cardboard box, the kind that appliances are shipped in. It can take some effort to track one down at your local department store, but it is well worth it. You can just leave the open-ended toys in a pile to be mined, or, if your children need a bit of encouragement, tell or read a story the day before, and then, that night, set up a scene with the new toys for your children to discover and explore the next day.

Part Three

Parenting Challenges: Ho Hum as a guide for discipline

Chapter Eight
Helping Children Understand
Consequences: Misbehavior and mistakes

In Part Two we looked at setting up a family environment that is likely to help with daily life, at work and at play. Yet even if we have a strong rhythm carrying us through transitions without heavy negotiation, and even if we have children who feel they create the household with us by taking on some shared chores, and even if there is play in which children can learn, thrive and be absorbed – even then, there will be challenges, instances of difficult behavior and times of conflict. Such problems are a normal part of parenting, indeed of being human. We can reduce them, but we can't eliminate them without all becoming robots. Our aim is to respond to conflict, not to eliminate it. Conflict has its own benefits and contributions to make, painful though they may be.

Problems, challenges and conflicts are where the principles of Ho Hum kick in. These are the moments when we need to:

1. Be calm;
2. Be confident in our parental authority;
3. Respond with actions and experiences rather than words.

Part Three contains many examples of Ho Hum in practice. It has stories of children making mistakes, throwing tantrums, refusing to cooperate, experimenting dangerously, fighting with each other, or challenging the boundaries they've been given, and it shows how these common problems can be met with calm authoritative parental action.

I will expand particularly on what kinds of actions and consequences are likely to be effective learning experiences for children: here you'll see how you can apply the third principle of Ho Hum in your daily family life.

Part Three applies Ho Hum to discipline for children, that is, it suggests ways of using Ho Hum to encourage positive behavior and discourage negative behavior. Discipline is not simply curbing a child's misbehavior or enforcing a set of rules, although it does include those. Discipline is modeling how to do the right thing, over and over again. It is taking the time to teach your child what *to* do, and that means doing it alongside him for as long as it takes. It is standing at the sink brushing your teeth while your child brushes his every morning and evening until he tells you he can do it on his own. Discipline is doing the household chores together instead of sending him to sweep the kitchen on his own while you are busy elsewhere. It is taking the time to be present with your whole self, not just your words. Discipline is establishing a daily rhythm and sticking with it, so that your child can rely on a familiar routine during the transitions of his day. It is restraining yourself from offering choices too early and being conscious of what you say. Discipline is sweating the small stuff: not letting his disrespectful words or behavior slide by in order to avoid a conflict. Discipline is not simply a response to misbehavior; it is the way you live your life. And it requires an immense quantity of self-discipline from us, the parents.

Think of discipline not as something to be applied to your children, but as an activity or practice of *yours*. It is your system for guiding and teaching, along the lines of a master and apprentice, but rather than imparting the skills of shipbuilding or running a restaurant kitchen, as a parent you are teaching your children how to live in the world as best you know how. You are showing them what to do and what not to do, and ultimately you are teaching them how to figure that out on their own.

Part Three starts here with a chapter about handling children's mistakes and misbehavior, and especially about the importance of children experiencing consequences when they misbehave. In order to learn, children need to have an experience that helps them change. Sometimes when parents talk about 'the consequences' – 'You must face the consequences!' – they mean punishment. Here, I don't mean punishment. I mean more literally that children need to learn that their actions have effects – they need to be confronted with the actual effects of their behavior. Parents have a guiding role in this. We sometimes need to make the connection between children's actions and the effects of those actions more obvious, and we sometimes need to step in and protect children if the consequences of their actions are dangerous. This is what we are aiming for when we act, as we're instructed in the third principle of Ho Hum.

Making Mistakes

There are three lessons that we must learn (or at least begin to learn, since we are never finished) in order to be prepared for adulthood:

1. All actions have consequences;
2. I am responsible for my actions;
3. I can correct my mistakes.

Children (and adults) will make a lot of mistakes during the process of learning these essential lessons about choices, actions and consequences (life!), and that is to be expected. Stumbling, backsliding and feeling lost or stuck are all part of the process of learning, and as long as children have the guidance they need, they will find their way back to the pathway of progress. **Problems with behavior are not a matter of a child being good or bad. They are a signal that the child still has some things to understand and learn, and that means that you still have some work to do to help him figure things out.**

As parents we fear our children's inadequacies as much, if not more, than our own, and this can make us quick to judge. What if they never learn? What if they never overcome their faults and weaknesses? What if they continue to make the same mistakes or worse? When our children misbehave, it can trigger the fear in us that the way they act now is a sign of who they are and who they will be. But labelling a behavior or a child as either good or bad – the two most basic categories – leaves us less able to take in further information, a broader perspective, or nuances. The relationship can get stuck dealing with this goodness or badness and the child will get stuck inside the label.

Ho Hum teaches us to focus on doing, not being: instead of getting caught up in what your children's behavior might say about who they *are*, try to keep your attention on what you and they need to *do*. Doing is where we can have influence, and steering away from conclusions about who they *are* allows children to make mistakes, learn and grow.

The question, then, for us parents is: *how* will we help our children to learn? When they have made a mistake or have misbehaved, what should they then be doing? What are the experiences we can give them, as distinct from the lectures full of words, which might lead to this behavior being less likely in the future?

I would suggest that what is most helpful is for children to feel the shift from guilt, shame or regret to the relief of making amends. Even with all of our practice and experience, we adults still make mistakes. When that happens, we recognize our errors and take measures to put things right. If we knock over our iced tea, we clean it up. If we back into someone's car in the parking lot, we pay for the repairs. And we reflect on our actions. The next time, we won't put our drink right next to our elbow. The next time, we won't try to pass a sippy cup to our child in the back seat when we are trying to pull out of a parking space. After our children have made a mistake, we can use Ho Hum to stay calm, step into our parental authority and then act in ways that encourage them in these processes: putting things right and reflecting on how it can be different in future.

All Consequences Are Not Equal

If you walk outside in a t-shirt when it is raining, you will get wet. If you wear a raincoat or bring an umbrella, you will stay drier. If you don't do the laundry, you will run out of clean clothes, and conversely, if you do your laundry, your clothes will be clean. If you drink a lot of sugary drinks, you will develop cavities in your teeth. If you stay up too late, you will be tired the next day. If you don't store food properly, it will spoil.

These are all forms of natural consequences. No one makes the results happen; they just do. No one designs the consequence in order to teach you a lesson or because you deserve it. The consequence will happen no matter what. The rain does not make you wet because you are bad. It simply falls, and you will get wet or not depending on your own decisions about what to wear.

Natural consequences can be very instructive, but some parents make the mistake of relying on them entirely, feeling that, as parents, they have no place interfering with their children's 'natural' learning process. But natural consequences are not all equally instructive.

The lessons that natural consequences have to offer can be lost for a number of reasons. Often the consequence is just too far removed from the child's action for him to experience it as the result of his choice. For example, the general feeling of unease and discomfort that a child experiences from eating a lot of junk food is too removed from the actual moments when he is eating for him to understand that there was a cause-and-effect relationship between his poorly chosen breakfast and his energy slump at mid-morning. **To be instructive, a consequence needs to be more immediate, and the younger the child, the more immediate the consequence must be in order for him to experience the connection.**

Natural consequences can be very harsh, even dangerous. Allowing a child to get a mouthful of cavities because he drinks a lot of sugary sodas will, possibly, get the point across (although in this case, he will have to rely on your or your dentist's say-so, since the connection will not necessarily be obvious), but it is a harsh way to learn the lesson. Even if he learns it well and never drinks another soda in his life, he will still suffer from the effects of the decisions he made while he was in the process of learning. It would be better for his parent to set some limits and to provide a more immediate consequence for exceeding those limits, one which would not involve permanent damage.

Natural consequences can play a useful part in your child's education, but they are not always adequate. Raising children is not a spectator sport. You are not there only to cheer your child along when he succeeds and commiserate when he suffers. **Your child needs guidance. Sometimes that happens naturally, but if the natural consequence is not instructive, you must provide one that is.**

An example: when natural consequences are not enough. If your young son touches something hot, he will feel the burning sensation and snatch back his hand. He may not know the meaning of the word 'hot,' but his body does, and it responds. He is unlikely to repeat the behavior, at least immediately. If, on the other hand, he slides his dinner plate off the edge of the table and watches it fall to the floor, he will understand that the plate falls and breaks and that the food scatters, but he will not necessarily know that this is an undesirable outcome. The ensuing chaos, with the dog responding valiantly to the call of duty, you exclaiming and grabbing a sponge and the food spreading into a fascinating pattern on the linoleum, may be significantly more entertaining and gratifying than simply eating the food would have been.

So while your child quickly comes to a basic understanding of gravity, like any true scientist, he will want to test the theory over and over again to confirm his expectations and to explore all the possible permutations. What is to stop him? He has no notions about the ethics of wasting food or of what it takes to replace a broken dish. Sure, he might feel hungry later because of the uneaten meal, but it is unlikely that he will connect that sensation to the earlier behavior. He is a creature of the present, and he learns from the immediate consequences of his actions.

It takes considerable maturity and life experience, certainly more than he has at this moment, to project into the future and weigh his possible choices against the outcomes he has experienced previously. In this case, the events that might teach him that his choice to knock his plate over is not acceptable are too far in the future for him to learn from them. You will need to provide a more immediate and instructive consequence.

Remember, children learn from what you do and from what they themselves do, not so much from what you say. In order for this child to learn that he must not dump his plate, you must do something that helps him to learn this. It is not enough to encourage positive behavior, although that should always be your first approach. You must also discourage (and redirect) negative behavior. A small boy who knocks his plate to the floor can be given plenty of opportunities to explore the nature of gravity in ways that don't cause problems, but his impulse to do it with his dinner *is* a problem, and because of that he needs to learn that there are limits to where and when he can perform those explorations.

In this case, if the child were very young, under three, you could calmly say, 'Dinner's over,' and help him down from his chair. If he were a little older, you could bring over two sponges, handing one to him and encouraging him to help you clean up – even if his efforts didn't amount to much at first. Should you fix him another plate? No. He was clearly not hungry enough to want to eat, and he does need to learn that if he dumps his food, that is the end of it for the moment. (Later if he is hungry he could have a snack. He is too young to connect his later hunger to his earlier action.)

Should you explain why dumping his dish is wrong? No. Words and the concepts they are meant to explain are not particularly effective and are a distraction from the real lesson at hand: dinner is over when you dump your plate. No judgment, no comment. It just *is*, undeniably and with absolute certainty, every time, just as the laws of physics are immutable and apply to all equally and without concern. Does this mean that he won't dump his plate again? Not necessarily. It might take a few times for him to learn. But as long as you are Ho Hum about it – calm, comfortable in your authority, clear and consistent in your actions (bringing dinner to an end) – he will figure it out.

There is a myth that small children cannot understand cause and effect. This is incorrect. It is true that they can't understand it if you explain it to them. If you were to say to your child, 'If you dump your plate, your dinner will be over,' rather than learning from your words, your child will have a strong impulse to test it out in practice. Children don't turn things over in their minds; they do it with their hands. Once he has dumped the plate, and dinner is over: 'A-ha,' he knows – because he has experienced it physically. So, in the interest of clarity and economy, it is better to skip the words and go right for the action.

You can help your child learn that all actions have consequences by responding to his misbehavior with Ho Hum: with calmness and clarity, comfortable authority and warmth, and, most especially, with an instructive experience.

I am Responsible for my Actions

In addition to learning that all actions – good, bad or neutral – are followed by the consequences of those actions, **all children must learn that they are responsible for their own actions. Children will** learn this lesson on their own, as long as parents don't provide the common roadblocks that prevent children from learning it: giving choices too early, or blaming and using punishment.

Giving Choices Too Early

Offering choices too early causes so many problems. Not only does it foster whiny children whose focus is primarily on satisfying their own wants, it also prevents children from learning to take any responsibility for their choices and actions. When you offer your young (under seven) child a choice, you may think that you are giving him, even teaching him, responsibility for his decisions. But small children do not learn the same way that adults do.

Children assume that if they are offered a choice, all the options are approved, and what they want will be provided. This is what the offer implies to them. If your child doesn't get what he wants, or if things go badly in some way, he will not look to his choice as the reason, but to you. To him, the outcome is your responsibility because you are the all-knowing parent – and he's not entirely wrong. By offering choices too early, you will teach your child that he is *not* responsible for either his choices or the consequences that follow. On the whole, make choices rather than offering them.

Blaming and Punishment

The goal is for your child to learn that he is responsible for his actions, and he can only do that is if it is safe for him to do so. A simple judgment-free statement of fact is all that is needed: 'That is a mess,' instead of 'You made such a mess. I can't believe you did that!' or some variation on that theme. Blaming connotes judgment, and, specifically, it connotes 'badness.' There is an implied threat behind that judgment: 'You are bad, and I disapprove of you.'

The fear that this judgment brings is, of course, the fear that you will no longer love your child and that, by being bad, he is not worthy of your love. This fear is not a great inducement for him to jump up and say, 'Yes, it was me. I dumped my plate off the table. I take full responsibility.'

While children learn that all actions have consequences through their bodies, through their physical experience of the events, they learn to take responsibility for their actions through their feelings – primarily their feelings of emotional safety. In order to take responsibility for his actions, including his mistakes, your child must feel safe doing so. Asking him to own a mistake when he also risks your love at the same time is asking too much.

Punishment is an extreme form of blaming. As such, it goes even further in preventing your child from learning the essential lesson that he is always responsible for his own actions. Punishment relies on the following assumptions: the behavior is bad, therefore the child is bad, therefore he must be made to feel badly so that he will not repeat the bad behavior and will also somehow, inside, become 'good.'

The idea behind punishing is that the child will learn to avoid the behavior in order to avoid the punishment. This can seem effective in the short term, but in the long term it encourages a child to feel less responsibility for his actions, not more. Avoiding misbehavior because he fears punishment is not real learning. If you are not there to dole out the punishment, there is nothing to stop your child from misbehaving again. When we use punishment, the motivation not to misbehave comes from without, not from within. Worse, your child fears you, and he fears further failure. Instead of reflecting on his choice and its repercussions for those around him – an essential ingredient if he is to develop self-discipline – his motivation becomes entirely oriented toward protecting himself from you. He will go to great lengths, not so much to avoid the misbehavior, but to avoid having you find out about it.

By judging him instead of instructing him about his choice, you may have temporarily stopped the misbehavior, but you have also created a situation in which you have overlooked your child's signals that he still has something to learn and needs your help and guidance, and, instead, you have taught him that you are not to be trusted. The next time he makes a mistake, instead of coming to you for help in dealing with it, he will hide it or try to deflect the punishment by lying or blaming someone else.

The feelings that punishment engenders in a child are not only counter-productive, they can be damaging as well. The fear of further punishment drives children to become wily, manipulative and secretive instead of forthcoming and honest. The judgment that the child is bad and that he must be made to feel badly leads the child to feeling ashamed – not of what he did, but of who he is. Punishment denies the full realities of the child's true self and seeks solely to eradicate the undesirable in him. This puts him in an impossible bind: he is who he is and no amount of punishment will change that.

He will either withdraw in defeat at this sentence of eternal inadequacy, or he will fight it, becoming angry. Instead of feeling remorse for his misbehavior, he will be nursing a desire for revenge. Feeling attacked, the child will not likely be concerned with his own actions, but will instead be focused on the injustice of yours. Instead of learning to take responsibility for his choices, a punished child denies them.

Punishment does not come from authority. It comes from power, and while it may curtail the immediate negative behavior, in the long run it sets the stage for a greater struggle between parent and child, one in which the child must either submit and lose himself, or try to undermine or wrest power away from her parent. Once this dynamic has been initiated by the parent using punishment, there are no longer any good choices for the child.

By judging the child as bad, the parent misses the opportunity to determine how and why the child came to make the mistake and to offer guidance where it was clearly needed. What wrong assumptions did he have? What does he need to understand? What tendency does he have that leads him to, say, dump his plate, and in what ways can the parent channel that tendency into something positive? Can the parent ennoble that aspect and at the same time limit it: teach him to not waste his dinner?

Giving choices too early, blaming and punishing all divert your child's attention from his responsibility for his actions. Concrete, physical consequences give your child the information that will help him understand the connection between his actions and the results of those actions. Without parental roadblocks in his way, your child will feel safe in making the connection between his choices and his actions. With that as a foundation, you can then show him what to do when he does make a mistake.

We Can Correct Our Mistakes

Truthfully, a mistake-free life is not to be sought after, since that would only occur if one were to stop learning and trying new things. As our children learn and grow, their expanding opportunities will bring potential for missteps, mistakes, and all-out failures, along with discoveries and successes. **In order that their mistakes do not permanently hinder them, children need lots of practice with the two basic elements for handling mistakes: action (making amends) and reflection.** Parents can help with these.

Action: Making Amends

A person can only fully make amends if he is willing to accept responsibility for his own actions. The importance of making amends is not just to restore wholeness to whomever was hurt or whatever was broken. It is to restore wholeness to the person who made the mistake, the one who caused the trouble in the first place. **Your child will learn to take responsibility for his mistakes if he learns that he can fix them by making amends. Model this process when you make a mistake. Help him do it when he makes a mistake.**

Here's an example: My son used to practice shooting hockey pucks in our garage. He had a net set up against the back wall in front of the shelving. While the storage boxes were dented in a few places, all went well until one day a wild ricochet put the puck through the only window on the side wall. I was inside and didn't hear the sound of the glass shattering, but Thomas came in looking sheepish and asked me if I would help him clean it up so that the cats wouldn't cut themselves. There wasn't a lot that needed to be said. After we swept up the shards, we went inside and called the window company. At that time, Thomas was about twelve and was still shy on the phone, so I agreed to make the call. He agreed to pay for the window.

The customer service representative asked, apparently as part of their quality control, why we needed to replace the window. When I mentioned that there was an incident involving a hockey puck and that my son would be covering the replacement cost, the man chuckled and told me he would call me right back. A short while later the phone rang, and he told me that he would be able to replace the window with a huge reduction in cost – he mentioned something about a 75 per cent employee discount and a hockey puck in his own past. While we waited for the new window, my son fitted cardboard into the empty space to keep out the snow, and dug deeply into his pockets and drawers to come up with the cash. The new window arrived, and the slate was finally clean – I suspect not only for my son, but for the man on the phone as well.

Thomas understood that it was his choice and his action that led to the broken window. He did not even try to weasel out of it based on the fact that I had moved the net over from its original place. He had not moved it back to where it should be for shooting pucks, and he knew it was his responsibility to do so. He was considerably anguished over the incident as well as being pretty irritated with himself. The admission by the company representative that he had done something similar as a youth made my son feel less foolish, or at least helped him feel less alone in his foolishness. Whatever he felt, my husband and I did not pile onto it by lecturing or complaining or in any way making a judgment. We simply helped him to fix it and move forward. And by fixing it, he was able to close the case. I am guessing that, for the man on the phone, there had not been such satisfactory closure – that his broken window had haunted him in some small way until he was able to make amends for whatever mistake he had made by helping our son make amends for his.

Teaching your child to make amends is not just your duty, it is a kindness. Whether he feels able to admit it openly or not, he will, on some level, know when he has caused harm, and if he doesn't know how to make amends, the burden of those mistakes will live with him forever. That is too much for anyone to carry. He must be given a means by which he can release that load in a responsible way, one in which wholeness is restored as much as is possible. Regret is a trap with iron jaws. Knowing how to make amends will free your child from its hold and will allow him to move forward. The focus shifts from the problem toward the solution: what a relief.

Let me be specific: the way to teach your child to make amends is relatively simple if you start early and start with action. Teach him to clean up and fix the messes that he makes. Don't worry so much, at this early stage, about the emotional fixes. Those are much more difficult and nuanced. By emphasizing the physical fixes, cleaning up spills and repairing or replacing broken items, you are laying the physical groundwork that will support later efforts to sort out and make amends for more interpersonal and emotional rifts. By learning it first with his body, your child will have the experience of being capable in a very concrete way, and he will also experience the sense of closure and relief that taking responsibility for his actions brings. This will encourage him later to try to work through more difficult problems: he will have a history of success based on effort, and he will have an understanding of the benefits of those efforts, for himself just as much as for the others involved.

In the meanwhile, you can be modeling for him the ways in which you make amends for mistakes that are more emotional.

The goal is for your child to empathize with the person he has wronged, so instead of focusing on your child: 'You hurt her feelings. Say you're sorry,' focus instead on the person who was hurt. Describe *the other child* and how she is feeling: 'Oh look, Sarah looks really sad. See how she stares at the ground?' and then figure out what to *do*: 'I wonder what we could do to make her feel better. Hmmm.' If your child *is* sorry, by all means have him say it. A sincere apology is very freeing and healing. An insincere one only pours salt in the wound. Forcing children to say 'I'm sorry' when they are not makes them resentful and less willing to accept responsibility for what they have done – and, even worse, you force them to lie, and that will cause a serious breach in their trust in you.

Use every opportunity you have to show your child how *you* make amends. The next time you snap at your husband, telling him that he always leaves the kitchen for you to clean up, make sure you apologize to him in front of your child: 'I am sorry. That really came out the wrong way. I can see that I upset you. What I meant to say is this: I am really tired right now. Would you help me with...' Apologize to your children, too, when you catch yourself yelling or otherwise doing something that hurts them. The bonus for us is that we can turn our mistakes into opportunities for teaching our children how to live life as imperfect beings. They will need to learn that, and the fact that we are imperfect makes us perfect teachers.

Reflection

Your child cannot move forward, or at least he cannot get far, if he resolves the problem he has caused only to repeat the original mistake over and over again. Some of the best lessons come from our mistakes, but the mistake is only the raw material; the learning comes from reflection upon that mistake. By thinking back over the situation to examine the choices he made and to consider what he was influenced by, he can determine where and how he went wrong, and he can then make a plan for the next time he is faced with something similar.

Small children cannot really engage in such reflection. They live too much in the present and learn almost entirely through their bodies, and it would be inappropriate to separate them from their world of now. Children under ten are too young to engage productively in reflection. They will, however, benefit as always from a good model: that would be you – again. When you make a mistake, not only can you make sure that your child sees you making amends, you can think out loud, talking yourself through your reflections on your choices and your plan for next time.

As your child nears adolescence, you can start to gently lead him through such a reflection, inviting his input. Once he is in his teens, it is appropriate, particularly when he has made a serious mistake, to require that he present you with his analysis of how he went wrong as well as a plan for the future. If you have given him plenty of modeling from the start and lots of opportunity to practice fixing his mistakes without the added burden of hasty judgment, he will likely come to you with his plan unasked, since he will want to show that he is indeed responsible and mature, despite a momentary slip.

I am sure that you are noticing some recurring themes. Respond to misbehavior with Ho Hum, that is, stay calm and don't react; step into your parental authority to find a way between abdicating all influence and attempting total control; and finally, look for the appropriate actions that will give your child a learning experience. Model the positive behavior yourself and treat misbehavior as an indication that your child needs guidance and practice, practice, practice. When your child misbehaves, it means only that you are not done yet. Another theme would be about how your child learns: first in his body with action, then with his feelings and his sense of connection and last, with his intellect, by thinking and reflecting. Action is the foundation of all learning, followed by feeling, with thinking being the final step. One is not more important or more valuable than another. It is just that action comes first.

Chapter Nine
Connecting Freedom and Responsibility:
Boundaries, rules, respect

One of the most important things we teach our children is that freedom comes, always and inherently, with responsibility. This is part of learning that all our actions have consequences, as we covered in the last chapter. I may be free to act, but I have to take responsibility for the outcomes of my actions. As children grow, they need more freedom and greater responsibilities, and it's our job as parents to gradually expand their boundaries. When we are faced with a situation in which our child has breached the boundaries and has not behaved responsibly, once we have found our calmness and have stepped into our parental authority, the action to take is to constrict that boundary. Rather than delivering a lecture, we want our child to *experience* the connection between freedom and responsibility: if she doesn't behave responsibly, her freedom shrinks.

Boundaries Expand and Contract

An example: When my son was young – about four years old – the world of the outdoors beckoned to him from the moment he woke until his little head hit his pillow at night. There were so many rocks and pebbles to be sorted and admired, so many holes to be dug. But I had things that kept me inside. What to do? The dog was deputized as babysitter and was sent out with him. An Australian sheep dog with more enthusiasm than focus, she greeted the arrival of anyone or anything new with a combination of loud, joyful barking and considerable bouncing around. With her on watch, it was unlikely that anything would sneak up unannounced, be it a moose or the UPS man, but she would be no help in keeping Thomas from straying out of the yard.

There was a boundary, the post-and-rail fence, but it would not keep him in unless he respected it. Would he do that? I thought it unlikely, but I was pretty sure that he could learn. So, he was sent out with instructions to stay inside the fence. We even walked around the whole perimeter, touching the fence. 'You may play outside as long as you stay inside this fence,' I said, and then I went in. But I didn't get to my work right away, or at least not entirely. As I moved through the house, I kept an eye and an ear out for him, keeping track of where he was.

Inevitably, he forgot about the boundary or disregarded it and was on the other side of the fence when I went to the window to check for the umpteenth time. So, out I went, Ho Hum, to get him. I pointed out to him where the fence was, and where he was in relation to it – just the facts – while reminding him that being outside alone to play meant staying inside that boundary. Taking his hand, we walked back into the house, where he played for the rest of the morning.

For the next several days, he had to wait for me to be free to come out with him if he wanted to go outside to play. No comment beyond a simple, 'You will have to wait until I am ready to go with you.' No judgment. That was just the way it was. **He stepped over the boundary, and as a result, that boundary became much smaller, not just for that moment, but for several days.**

In fact, the boundary remained in that constricted state until he accepted it with grace, with no whining, pleading or carrying on. There was a way to show that he had learned from his mistake, that he understood what had happened and why, and that he was willing to accept the consequence – the tighter boundary. That acceptance indicated a step forward, letting me know that it was time to try again.

Out he went once more, with the dog circumscribing him with ecstatic leaps (there was no question who suffered the most from the confinement), the lesson fresh in his memory. This time, he understood it on a physical level, which is really the only level for such a young child, and so equipped, he managed to stay inside the fence. I checked regularly, but he never crossed that line again. It had been the same with my daughter earlier.

The only real way they had of knowing that the boundary was there was to test it in a concrete, physical way. **Children don't test boundaries because the boundaries are unjust. They test them in order to know them. It is the only way they can.** Like Peter Rabbit, who comes home from the forbidden garden and is relieved to take himself and his upset tummy to his safe bed, children are relieved to know that the boundary is there. 'Are you paying attention to me?' they wonder. 'Do you care enough to get up and come get me? Am I worth it?' They want to know.

They won't have to test every boundary to learn to respect them, especially when you address the crossing of the early physical boundaries with Ho Hum. These simple lessons lead your children to understanding the connection between their actions and the consequences that follow them, as well as the relationship between freedom and responsibility. They will understand that their level of freedom, their boundary, hinges not on your whim or on their ability to wear you down, but on their level of responsibility. **So when they desire more freedom, a wider boundary, they know that the way is not through rebellion, not through overt and covert forays beyond the limit, but instead the way is through *earning*: showing that they are capable, responsible and respectful.** In other words, through showing that they are ready.

Ideally, you will be able to expand the boundaries over time, giving your maturing child more room, more leeway and more options as she shows that she is ready. There will be moments when you will contract those boundaries, when your child has stepped too far over, or when she has lost herself and needs more support (a tighter boundary can be a real relief). Start small and expand gradually, making adjustments along the way.

It is very hard to teach an older child to respect boundaries when she has not learned them as a young child because there is so much for her to unlearn: the primary issue being that she will have learned that freedom is *not* connected to responsibility. She will feel entitled to freedom and will resent you and anyone else who expects her to earn it. Make the effort at a younger age if you can.

When you do contract your child's boundary in response to her breaking of the boundary, don't designate a time frame. **The boundary stays contracted until she accepts the restriction with grace and good will. She must show that she can be responsible in order to earn the expansion of her boundary. She is not serving a term, but is, instead, experiencing the consequence of not respecting a reasonable boundary.** If she wants to change that boundary, there is a responsible way to ask you about that. Breaking it is not that way. The duration of the restriction depends entirely on her.

It is not the severity of the restriction that matters, but the certainty. You are not trying to induce enough suffering that your child avoids the behavior. You are simply helping her make the connection between her behavior and the consequences of that behavior. People don't generally learn well when they are under emotional duress. Your child may, in fact, be upset when her boundaries are contracted, but that is a whole different world from the fear, anger and resentment that punishment incurs. If an emotional storm ensues when you withdraw a freedom and contract a boundary, handle it as you would any tantrum.

It is important not to give in to breaches of a boundary, or you will teach that pushing at boundaries is an effective means of gaining greater freedom. Your child will learn she can get what she wants through manipulation rather than through responsible and respectful action.

Retracting freedom differs from, say, 'grounding' because it is more specific to the particular boundary that has been breached, and its aim is not punishment, but a connecting of freedom and responsibility.

Here's an example to clarify this: Our neighbor's son once drove into a vehicle that was stopped in front of him. This happened because he was driving too fast, and he had a friend in the car, which halves a teenager's ability to focus. The boy also had another minor fender bender while talking on his cell phone. It was inconvenient for my neighbors to drive their son where he needed to go, which would have been my first choice for a response. They did have the option of limiting him to driving alone, and also withholding the cell phone. They chose, instead, for their son to do some extra chores to make amends for the stress and hardship his bad choices had placed on the rest of the family. This, unfortunately, did nothing to improve his driving habits, as there was then a third driving incident, although thankfully it was minor.

The penance may have reconciled the balance sheet in terms of my neighbor's aggravation, but it did nothing to limit the boy's freedom to drive. To the teenager, the price of doing a few extra chores was obviously worth the risk of driving while distracted. If done in lieu of payment for the damage on the car, the extra chores might have been appropriate, but alone, without the contraction of the boundary, there were not enough to make the teen take his driving responsibilities seriously.

Restricting your child's freedom usually involves more supervision from you. Make sure that you are willing and able to follow through. Parents often prefer other consequences because they are easier (they think), but putting the time in up front will pay dividends later on.

Teenagers' Freedom and Rebellion

Often parents assume that because teenage rebellion is common, it is inevitable, even a milestone. As long as parents buy into this assumption, they will not see how they set the stage for rebellion, nor will they understand that it is a poor substitute for the teen's true objective.

Ideally (and I say 'ideally' knowing that none of us will ever be perfect), as our children grow and mature, we will build a foundation of trust. We will expand their choices and boundaries when appropriate, and we will guide them towards responsibility and the freedom that springs from it. There will be times when the forward motion along this continuum will be temporarily stalled, when a bad choice or momentary act of resistance requires a restriction of freedom and choice. A little bit of testing to check the boundaries is to be expected. This is the way teenagers get their bearings and reassure themselves that you are paying attention, that you care enough to hold the line.

The key is to make sure that you are both moving generally in the right direction along the progression from dependence, protection and guidance towards independence, freedom and responsibility – that you, the parent, are in fact releasing your child, however incrementally. It is our job to gauge how quickly we move with our children along this continuum, and we must use every tool available to us: observation, intuition, experience, and, when all else fails, hindsight.

It is not a bad thing for teenagers to have to occasionally petition for an expansion of their freedom, making a reasoned (and often impassioned) plea for the consideration of their perspective. You would do well to hear it with respect and to treat it generously, finding even some small way to extend a 'Yes.' There may be a time when you offer a freedom first, judiciously gambling on the chance that the teenager will rise to the occasion and display a greater maturity. These occasional petitions for freedom are entirely different from wholesale opposition to your authority, where teens seize freedom before they possesses the maturity and responsibility to handle it. When this happens, it is easy to rationalize the behavior as typical of all teenagers. It is simple to lay the blame on the rebellious adolescent. It is simple but wrong.

This sort of opposition and defiance is the predictable result when parents reverse direction or refuse to move past a certain point on the progression toward allowing their child freedom and responsibility. Sometimes a parent is so strict and domineering that she is unwilling to recognize and connect with the emerging self of her child, and she controls every choice so tightly that the growing teenager is kept in a perpetual state of forced childhood with its concomitant dependence. Unable to gain freedom and independence in a responsible way, the teen seeks it by going to extremes. The teen has no choice but to revolt against the complete obstruction to her progress.

Parents who would pride themselves on being more open-minded and more sensitive to their child's emerging self may be surprised to find themselves in exactly the same boat as the more repressive parents. These parents, either through a lack of will or by a conscious desire to avoid 'crushing the child's spirit,' may have given their children lots of freedom in their early years: lots of choices and few boundaries. This apparent freedom and independence can seem delightful when the children are young, but as they reach teenagehood, it presents a problem. The children are accustomed to making their own choices and behaving as they like, and when the consequences of this become more serious and unpalatable, they don't have the safety net of consistent guidance to fall back upon.

The parents must now try to exert influence without having built a foundation of trust or establishing their authority. Having left the gates wide open, they now try to swing them shut by significantly restricting their teenager's freedom in an effort to limit the bad choices. The teen recognizes that this reversal is not as it should be, and she rebels. Fundamentally, she is right: at this stage, she should be moving forward in the direction of increased freedom and responsibility. But because her parents gave her the former without the benefit of the latter, she has not learned that the two must go hand in hand. Her rebellion, unlike that of the child of the repressive parent, is not based on actual repression, but the impression of it, and it is her permissive parents who have created that impression.

There is another phenomenon that leads to rebellion: when parents hurry their children, encouraging them to look, act and feel much older than they really are. These parents misunderstand the nature of real independence. A child who is truly independent is allowed to be dependent and is given all the support and guidance she needs. When the child is ready, she steps out on her own, choosing to take on challenges.

Children who are left to their own devices too early will often manage anyway. They can be remarkably resourceful and resilient, but this is coping with abandonment. It is not independence. Parents who thrust their children forward will find that it is hard to reverse course when their child's 'maturity' proves to be superficial and gets the best of them.

The true objective of teenagers is to mature into capable adults. When parents thwart that objective by holding them back or pushing them ahead before they are ready, teens respond by rebelling. This in itself is not a particularly mature response, and as such, it represents yet another obstacle to reaching their objective, which only creates more frustration for everyone. It becomes a self-perpetuating cycle. If this does happen, it is up to the parent to find a way to step out of it, to find some way of recognizing and honoring the underlying impulse toward maturity, even if it has manifested in a way that looks like the exact opposite.

Teenagers want to be trusted with freedom. They want to be capable of shouldering responsibility. They want to test their own theories and develop their own perspectives. They want to meet challenges and do it with flair. They want to discover and become themselves. What could be more bold? What could be more revolutionary? They don't need to rebel in order to do that.

Consequences When Rules are Broken

What sorts of actions can we take when our children break or disobey rules, failing to heed the boundaries of safety or respect? We can be sure that children need clear, specific rules and boundaries, and they need us to consistently maintain them when they are broken. If you have laid the groundwork with lots of modeling, with strong rhythm and with clarity about your own authority, you will find that your boundaries can be very simple and quite limited, and those are the best kind.

Rules and boundaries should not be a matter of interpretation or opinion. Fuzziness invites challenge. A clear rule or boundary is specific and concrete. My son was very handy, always building and constructing, and hence he wanted access to the tools. We wanted to encourage his explorations but didn't want him to get hurt. So when he was young, instead of telling him in a general way to 'be careful' or 'use good judgment,' we were specific: he was allowed to use any tool at any time, except for the power tools, which were forbidden – and that meant any tool that needed to be plugged in. He cut himself once or twice, certainly less than I did in the same amount of time, and proceeded with more caution after doing so. As he matured, the rule changed, reflecting his growing level of ability and responsibility, and he was then only required to make sure that an adult was home and awake before using the power tools. The line was always very clear, and he never crossed it. Had he done so, his access would have been restricted, and he knew it. He enjoyed the freedom that he had, and he wanted to keep it.

Where safety is concerned, I believe it is possible to be too protective. Do all that you can to protect children from the actions of others, but give them as much room as your pounding heart can manage when it comes to their own actions. I insist that my children wear helmets when they ride a bike, but I don't dictate the size of the jump that they construct. There are limits: the blow torch is locked away, for example, and they must construct the jumps from scratch instead of using existing structures like, say, the barn roof. This early connection to and balance between limit and freedom in their physical safety translates later to less tangible situations involving emotional or even financial safety.

But it is normal for children to break rules and boundaries from time to time. Ho Hum will help you respond when they do. The lifeblood of the town we lived in was the tiny ski hill right beside it. With a pleasantly low-rent and homey atmosphere, it was the place to run into your neighbors, your plumber and the city court judge. A bargain-basement-cheap season pass gave one the opportunity to go anytime for as long or as short as one pleased, and young children went for free. So our children learned to ski early, and as you would expect, they took to it easily and naturally, except for one part: the lift. Our daughter had no problem with it, but it became a real issue with our son. The lifts were ancient and rudimentary, and they often broke down, leaving whoever was riding them to sit, swinging from the cable, until the operators got them going again.

One day, this happened while my son and I were on the lift. Usually we passed the time by swinging our legs, clapping and singing rounds with the folks in the chairs nearby in an effort to pass the time as well as to keep warm. This time my normally cheerful boy became possessed by a foul mood, and with a deep frown on his face, he slid down and down in his seat – which meant that he was slipping farther and farther underneath the one bar that was supposed to hold him in. As he squirmed, I told him that it was not safe – the ground was fifty feet below – and that he must sit back in the seat: our one rule. That only seemed to make him more determined to squirm farther down.

Unwilling to let the natural consequence take its course, I hauled him up by the armpits and put my arm across his chest, locking him into his seat, gently but with absolute firmness. I was not going to let him fall as he seemed bent on doing. Without another word, we sat there in our silent struggle until the lift bumped, lurched and got moving. We got off at the top and skied down the hill, where I proceeded to unbuckle us from our skis. 'What are we doing?' my son asked.

'Going home,' I replied. And home we stayed for the rest of the season, which at that point was only a few weeks. When my husband and daughter bundled up each weekend and headed out, my son and I stayed home. No comment. No judgment. I was not willing to take him on the lift if he would not abide by the simple rules of safety. Stepping over that boundary meant that the boundary was, in this case, pulled in quite a bit. It is not fun to wrestle with a four-year-old boy when you are fifty feet about the ground with one small bar across your waist. I simply wasn't going to do it again. And I didn't have to. The next year we tried again, and no matter how long we had to wait, he followed the basic safety rules. The action I took gave him a powerful experience of direct consequence.

Rules and boundaries work best when children see that they are consistently applied. A high school teacher once told me this **story about consistency:**

It was her rule that all students must be in her class on time. When the bell rang, she locked her door, and any latecomers would miss class and have to make it up. Throughout the year, for various reasons, many of the students found themselves arriving to class late and found the door locked. There were two students who, in addition to being popular and at the top of the class, had been on time every day. She described how, on the last day of school, as the bell rang, she strode over to the door, preparing to turn the lock as usual, when she noticed that her two star pupils were not in class. She hesitated momentarily. Should she give them an extra minute? They had been so responsible all year, and they really did contribute so much to the class.

Unknown to her, all eyes were on her hand: would she lock the door or not? Before the last echo of the bell died away, she sighed, flipped the lock and turned... to a standing ovation. In fact, the 'good' students were standing right outside the door. It had been a test for the teacher, cooked up by the whole class, to see if she really would apply the rule consistently, no matter who broke it. She passed a test that shockingly few other adults would have. Already a favorite teacher, she earned something more precious to her that day: their trust and their respect.

Notice this was the students' test for her. What mattered to them most, what they needed in order to trust and respect her fully, was consistency. They *wanted* her to pass this test. From the students' perspective, consistency equals justice and the authority who applies boundaries consistently merits trust and respect. And the opposite is true as well. Children, and teenagers in particular, do not trust or respect adults who have no expectations of them, who do not set boundaries for them, and who do not maintain those boundaries consistently. If your child crosses a boundary, don't make excuses for her. Enforce the boundary – she wants you to.

Resistance

Here's another story about lateness that indicates action you can take if your children are dragging their feet, refusing to cooperate or resisting your authority. Delaying or refusing when the family tries to leave the house is a frustrating form of resistance. When my daughter was about ten, she was taking dance lessons in town, and every afternoon I would drive her there. She always packed up her bag and got herself ready to go while I helped her younger brother. But one day I found myself sitting in the car with the engine running, waiting for her. And the next day, it was the same, and the next day.

I knew she knew how to get ready since she had been doing it for years. I went back to 'doing with' but this only seemed to make her slow down even more. Boy! Did she know how to push my buttons! I asked her if she was having trouble in class, but she indicated that she was enjoying it. So then, since I couldn't actually *make* her move any faster, I had to decide what I was willing and not willing to do. I was willing to take her to dance like I always did, but only if she were ready on time. I told her, 'If you are in the car at 4:30, we will go.'

The next day, she came running out the door in a flurry of tears and flying hairpins, just as I was walking back in. She missed class that day. Was she upset? Yes, momentarily. But the choice had so obviously been hers, and my lack of blaming and lecturing and my commiseration with her disappointment left the responsibility squarely at her own feet. The next day she was ready on time, with a few minutes to spare, and it was never an issue again. Her dance class was a privilege, not an entitlement. If she had really needed help getting ready to go, I would have given it to her. She didn't. She was testing the boundary, and I am not particularly sure why she chose lateness, other than, perhaps, that it was a surefire way to get my goat.

Our children do know how to push our buttons. It is not that they are manipulative or diabolical, although when they do it, it can feel that way. It is simply that they are connected to us. They know us so sometimes they push. And they do so, hoping that we will act like the mature adults we are and hold the line without adding to the drama. They throw down the gauntlet to test our authority, not our patience. When they do that, it is because they are feeling vulnerable, not strong. They need us to show them that we are noticing them and that we love them enough to act. Words just don't cut it.

What if your child is dragging her feet about getting ready to go somewhere that is not her choice – say, school? That is tougher, for sure. If there isn't something she's afraid of or worried about, if she simply doesn't like school and is hoping to get out of a few minutes, you might talk with the teacher to see if there was a way for her to spend time in the classroom after school that equaled the time missed in the morning. We all have to do things that we don't want to do. Make her foot-dragging a waste of *her* time.

Rudeness and Disrespect

If we do not expect children to be respectful and if we don't guide them, always, back to the path of respect when they have wandered off, they will find that their opportunities to learn respect become quite limited as they mature. A child who is disrespectful becomes an adult who is disrespectful. Unfortunately, it is not enough to model respect. There are too many others in the world who model disrespect, and every child will try her hand, not because she is 'bad,' but because she is curious and she is an imitator. When she tries it out, your response will send her a message.

So what can you do when your child does say something rude? If you overlook it, your child has no way of knowing the difference between what you are ignoring and what you are allowing. Try redirecting. This is especially helpful when children are young. **Treat the rudeness as the mistake it is, and suggest what would be a more acceptable way of saying what she is trying to say.** If your child says, 'That's gross,' when passed a bowl of coleslaw, you can say, 'How about: *No, thank you,*' or 'Try this: *I don't care for any.*' Don't force her to repeat the better option after you, just let her know what it is, without judgment but also with a quiet assurance that she will pick it up.

In this way, you are modeling and you are 'doing with,' and at some point you and she will both be clear that she knows what to say. The age at which that point arrives will depend on how much guidance she has had, so setting it is impossible, but it will likely not be before she is five or six and probably not after age eight or ten.

In the event that an older child – one who knows better – speaks disrespectfully, you can simply call her attention to her error: 'That is disrespectful.' Then you can sincerely invite her to 'Try again,' and sincerely means not gritting your teeth while you say it or doing anything that would imply: 'Or else...' You are aiming more for something like, 'Oh, whoops, that didn't come out right. Why don't you try again?'

Let her know that you want to hear what she has to say. Sometimes you might still need to suggest, quite earnestly, how she might say it. She may be so lost in her grumpy world that she literally can't come up with the right words. But she needs to graciously accept the opportunity to correct herself. She must learn that she can broach any topic with you, but that she must do so in a normal, respectful tone.

If your child will not accept the opportunity to fix her mistake right away, then the action you can take that is a useful, instructive consequence is a separation in physical space between her and the other people present. That could mean just having a seat to the side or being escorted (kindly but firmly) to the living-room sofa if she insists on being rude at the table. 'You are welcome to come back as soon as you are ready to be respectful,' you can say. I often offer, 'Let me know if there is anything I can do to help you sort it out.' There is no anger on your part. You don't love her the less for it, but equally she cannot participate if she is going to be rude.

Let her know by your demeanor that you want her back. We all get grumpy, sure, but that does not mean that we get to inflict that grumpiness on everyone else. The first step is for her to literally take a step away to gain some perspective and understanding.

This is not a 'time out,' when she is supposed to feel isolated and in doing so, somehow be motivated to reflect on her misbehavior. No, this is just reality. She doesn't need to feel bad, and she will probably not use this time to reflect, although she might do so later, if you can hold onto your Ho Hum. In fact, **she can do whatever she needs to do to help herself feel better, and as soon as she is ready to be respectful, she is welcome to return. Don't force an apology. Don't force her to 'Try again' again.** It is actually embarrassing to be disrespectful. Instead of dwelling on it and risking her getting grumpy all over again, let her return and move forward by being respectful from that moment on.

If disrespect or rudeness happens away from home, and your child refuses to 'Try again,' an immediate return home is ideal. Don't be deterred by the inconvenience of doing this. If you act clearly and calmly to indicate that you will limit her access to the public until she shows that she is able to be more responsible with her words, she will very quickly find that disrespect hurts her more than you – as in truth it does. While she will still slip (we all do), she will readily correct herself the next time when you remind her, 'Try again.'

If your teenagers – or younger children – are rude while in front of friends, deal with it, but do so without humiliating them. Let's say, for example, that as you pull up in the car to pick up your teenage son and his gear, he says to you in that how-could-you-be-so-stupid tone, 'No, Mom, why are you stopping there? I can't open the trunk.' Instead of yelling at him through the passenger window, as you probably feel like doing, take a deep breath – Ho Hum – and call him around to your window to tell him, 'That was disrespectful. Try again.'

He will understand that while you are not going to tolerate his rudeness for one minute no matter who is out there being impressed by his display of bravado, you will also allow him to fix it with you privately, in a way that allows him to save face. Discipline is for guidance, not for humiliation. Elsewhere, you might ask him to step into another room with you, but make sure that you correct the rudeness right away. Don't wait until you get home or until it is more convenient.

Restaurants, churches, weddings and other public gatherings are the very last places you want to work out your issues with basic manners or boundaries. **If you have a disaster at a restaurant or other public place, that doesn't mean that you need to work on your child's manners while you are at restaurants or out and about. It means that you need to work on your child's manners and boundaries at home.** Be willing to leave. Your child is not ready for this; there is more work to do. Ho Hum. No comment. No judgment.

Chapter Ten
Tantrums

Ho Hum Meets the Tantrum

There are two kinds of tantrums, and you treat both the same way.

The first kind is a variation on this scenario: You have been running errands all afternoon with your toddler. He has been in and out of his car seat a handful of times, and you are at the last stop – the grocery store. Your son is showing signs of having had enough, but you are low on milk and out of bread completely. You just have to get through this one last errand and then you are home free. You head in and pull out a cart, but he clings to you, not wanting to sit. For the millionth time, you wish for that third hand as you try to cram a dripping head of lettuce into a plastic bag that is hermetically sealed at both ends. You manage, hiking him higher up on your hip as you head for the dairy aisle, but it is not your lucky day. There are only two more items to go, but your child has reached the end of his rope and bursts into tears, wailing loudly. People turn around and stare as you try to murmur comforting noises, but your son is past the point of no return. The day has been too long, the lights in the store are too bright, and the music and crowds are just too much. His back arches and his face turns bright red. He is overcome and howls in misery.

The second kind is something like this: A few aisles over, another mother is shopping with her youngster. She pauses to scan the upper shelves, and her son spots a colorful box of cereal and says, 'Mommy, I want that.' Mom, still looking elsewhere, says, 'Not today,' and pushes the cart farther along. The boy leans around his mother, reaching for the coveted box. 'But I want it! I want it,' he cries as he tries to get out of the cart. Mom, embarrassed and exasperated, says, 'We don't eat that kind. Here, why don't you help me pick out some apples,' but her son is determined. Suddenly, and for reasons he doesn't understand, getting that box is a matter of life and death. His chin quivers, he looks up at his mother with pleading puppy eyes, and when that doesn't bring the desired result, he arches his back and lets loose, keeping an eye on that box of cereal as his mother wheels the cart out of the aisle.

Both of these children are having tantrums. They are overwhelmed by their discomfort, and they are expressing themselves in the only way they know how. The first one's resources had been entirely depleted by the time he got to the grocery store. Overtired and stretched too far, he fell apart. The second child might also have been tired before he got to the store. Or not. Regardless, he decided that he wanted something, and when he didn't get it, he hoped to change his mother's mind by appealing to her sense of pity, and when that failed, the child resorted to the time-honored persuasion technique of throwing a full-blown tantrum. When a child has a tantrum, there can be both needs and wants at work.

How can you tell the difference? Luckily, you don't have to, because you treat them both the same way. While the motivations for the tantrum may vary, the source is always the same: discomfort. And that makes your job surprisingly simple (which is not the same as easy, but sometimes we have to settle for what we can get). **What do you do? Two things: attend to the discomfort by responding calmly and with warmth, and then carry on.** That is to say, you use Ho Hum: you stay calm and maintain your parental authority, then you act by comforting and, when the emotions have settled, your child's experience is that you continue with your activity.

Attending to the Discomfort

Children have myriad needs that change over time, from clean diapers to driving instruction, and it is our job to meet those needs as best we can. There are whole books out there, along with countless other resources, including the sum of the memories and life-experience of all the grandmas and grandpas of the world, which can tell us how to attend to our children's basic needs (they will contradict each other, and that means that, in the end, we have to figure it out for ourselves). Sometimes we miss something, or we forget, or we are too tired or we simply don't have access to the necessary resources. Each parent does the best she can and makes adjustments as she is able, but none of us will get it right every time, and as long as we get it right most of the time, there is no harm done.

When a child is having a tantrum, it is always worth tracing backwards from it to determine what might have set it off. Is he hungry or tired or overstimulated or understimulated? And it is always worth making an adjustment, if possible, so that the need can be better met in the future. For example, the mother of the first child above might consider spreading out her errands over a period of days, if possible, so that her little one wouldn't be so overwhelmed. She could make sure that her child has adequate snacks to get him through a long afternoon, and a good nap never hurts. Those considerations and adjustments can go a long way toward preventing the next tantrum, but what can she do right *now* with this tantrum?

A child who is having a tantrum needs human warmth. Even the child who flails his arms and legs and says terrible things in an apparent effort to drive away anyone who comes near, needs this warmth. He needs your calm presence. He needs your touch. He needs to be carried – literally, and also in the sense that you manage things for him in that moment.

And he needs your patience. He needs you there, holding things together, reliably and confidently, at a time when he has gone all to pieces. It may take him a while to come around. Can he trust that you will be there when he does, with warm, gentle hands that hold him snugly, firmly, but not too tightly, even if he is lashing out? Can he trust that you will be there with kind eyes that look into his without frustration or disgust, that know the shape of his whole being and have not forgotten it, even if he has? And, most of all, can he trust that, when he has finally come around, the world will still be the same?

While everything became unmoored inside him, did the world shift in some great seismic event? For his sake, it had better not. That would be too frightening. And this is why, after attending to his discomfort while he is in the midst of his tantrum, it helps him if you carry on as usual when he is done.

Carry On

Take a moment – take several even – to catch your own breath and allow your child to come back to the world. But when he has been released from the tantrum, his head resting on your shoulder, his breathing back to normal with a big sigh and no more hiccups, it is time to gently pick up where you left off. If you have returned home from the grocery store, that doesn't mean jumping in the car to get what you left sitting in the cart. It means carrying on with whatever comes next in your day. Your physical activity, your forward momentum, shows your child that while a tantrum may consume him temporarily, it will not consume you.

Your child needs to know that his moment of distress will not fundamentally alter the course of events. He will be reeling from it for a while. His senses will be tender and exposed: raw. Instead of putting all of your focus on him at this time, give him some space to let his senses scab over – not space in the sense of putting him down and leaving him alone, but space from your focused attention. Let him gather himself while you step back into the flow, folding him into the rhythm of the world as you carry him along. This is the reassurance that he needs.

But what about the child who throws a tantrum in the hopes of getting what he wants, or who, on not getting it by other means, is so upset that he is tipped over the emotional edge and falls apart? How should you respond to him? No differently. Attend to the discomfort that he feels, for it is genuine, regardless of the cause, and when the tantrum is over, carry on.

The child who has a tantrum because he doesn't get what he wants needs to learn a fundamental truth, but he can't learn it when he is upset. Help him through the emotional roller-coaster ride, and then, by getting back to things. By simply picking up where you left off when the tantrum started, you will be teaching him what he needs to know: wants are not needs. He, too, must learn that his distress will not change events.

If you were to give him what he wanted in order to avoid the embarrassment and inconvenience of dealing with his emotional response, you would be teaching him a rather dangerous lesson: that not getting what he wants is truly a crisis that must be avoided at all costs. Obviously, if you will do anything to head off the tantrum, it must be unbearable to you, and what is unbearable to you must be even more so to him.

This response – attending to your child's discomfort and then carrying on – is applicable no matter how old your child is. The toddler who fussed because he doesn't get the asked-for lollipop and the teenager who shouts and cries that you don't love him when you refuse permission for a social event both need the same thing: for you to attend to his emotional and/or physical discomfort with warmth and kindness, and when he has settled down, for you to carry on as usual.

Ho Hum is Not Easy

You will notice that the key to responding to tantrums and all forms of resistance is your ability to have a calm presence, in other words, to have Ho Hum. This is hard to do. That is an understatement. I don't have to tell you how hard that is. Even if you understand the principles of Ho Hum, of listening to and understanding your emotions, of being confident in your authority, of responding with action, Ho Hum is still very difficult. But practice does make it easier.

And – call it irony, divine justice or whatever you want – we are all given opportunities to practice it until we get it right. It is, in that way, self-correcting. When we respond before we have reached Ho Hum, we rarely achieve true and lasting resolution to the issue or problem at hand. When we respond with anger or impatience, we most often are punting the problem down the road, where it patiently waits and steps out to meet us again when we finally catch up. Be grateful for this: that the problem will lurk out there, waiting for you. Why be grateful? Because it means that no matter how you bungle something, and we all do, you will get another chance to do better.

While Ho Hum requires us to act, it does not require us to always act immediately. There will be times when your child has pushed a boundary or pushed one of your buttons in a way that makes you so upset or angry that you just cannot achieve Ho Hum. You cannot get to a place of calmness. If you can catch yourself before you act (or react), wait. Yes, let it go for a moment. You can tell your child that you will respond later, to let him know that you have taken note of the issue and recognize the problem, but that you will be addressing it later. **Give yourself time and space to cool down before you respond.**

Get some space. Talk it out with your spouse or a friend. Pack up and go home if need be. That old saying 'Don't go to bed angry' is wrong in this case. No problem will be solved when emotions are high. **Take the time to sleep on it – this can do wonders.** You will find that the next morning you will have much more perspective. You may still feel the presence of the anger or the guilt, fear and hurt, but in your sleep, you will have sat down with them all at the proverbial kitchen table and will have heard what your emotions are telling you, and in the morning, you will be better informed and more able to proceed with more balance.

Chapter Eleven
Lying and Trust

Lying is one of those parental challenges in which it takes particular exertion to focus on what you and your child need to *do*, rather than slipping into panic about who your child *is*. But, as with other challenges, Ho Hum is your lifeline here. Before we look at what to do and where to focus, though, I also suggest that you reduce the instances when you might suspect your child of lying by not offering her opportunities to lie.

In a situation where you think your children have done something wrong, asking them to tell you the truth may seem like the obvious way to teach them to be honest and responsible for their choices, but in practice this approach is riddled with pitfalls. You may be disappointed in the results. More significantly, you may sacrifice the ultimate goal: trust.

Am I suggesting you accept lies? Absolutely not. It is not that children and teens should not be responsible for their actions or words. It is that we adults need to do a better job at guiding them to be truthful, and ultimately, trustworthy (an even higher goal in my mind), and, as counter-intuitive as it may seem, we don't do that by asking them to tell the truth. There is nothing inherently wrong with telling the truth – that is indeed what we are striving for. It is the *asking* that is so problematic.

Unintended Consequences

Let's say that you leave your change in a bowl on your dresser, and one day you notice that it has disappeared. You didn't actually see who took it but obviously someone did, so you ask your child if she took it. She says no. If you decide to believe her, there is always the possibility that she is lying. Do you really want to give her the opportunity to lie? If she gets away with it, she may be awfully tempted to do it again. If she is caught later with jangling pockets, she may be filled with remorse, but it is also possible that it will only motivate her to do a better job covering her tracks next time.

On the other hand, if she is, in fact, *not* guilty, will you be able to wholeheartedly accept her version of events, or will you harbor doubts? If you doubt her, she will surely feel it, and she will be confused: what was the point of telling you the truth when you did not fully believe her?

Have you noticed that we only demand that children tell us the truth when we know or suspect that they are guilty of something? If you walk into your child's room to find finished homework stacked neatly on her desk, you are unlikely to say 'Tell me the truth about what's been happening here this evening.' We usually only ask children if they are guilty once we already think they are. There is a discernible pattern, and they will pick up on it quickly – making their answering even harder.

I once confronted my young daughter about some suspected transgression, my stomach in knots because I wanted her to admit her wrongdoing, and I anticipated failure (a denial, a lie). In that state of mind, I would be suspicious of a denial, whereas an admission would leave me feeling more certain and therefore more comfortable. If she had done something bad, at least she could redeem herself somewhat by telling the truth, right? I was more upset about the prospect of a lie than I was about the actual transgression (which, of course, I no longer remember).

As I waited, my daughter was looking at me anxiously, a tumult of fear and confusion on her face as she groped for the right answer. What was the right answer? She was trying to figure out what I wanted to hear. Should she tell me she was guilty, even if she weren't, if that was what I was waiting for? The implication was that the truth and the right answer might not always be the same. And if she was guilty, she risked disappointing me no matter whether she told me of her wrong or lied about it.

How is a child supposed to navigate such a complicated maze? How is she to choose? How could she trust me when I was expecting her to make what was, for her, an impossible choice? **'Telling the truth' is riskier and more complicated for children than we may realize.**

The truth, the whole truth and nothing but the truth can be pretty elusive, even for adults. We have a whole trial system set up to determine this, and a jury is made up of twelve adults because we know that very often there are nuances to truth, varying stories even among eye-witnesses, and different perspectives. It can take a lot of sorting. When we ask our children for the truth, it seems so simple and obvious: just tell it. But it is not as simple as that, and they feel frightened and alone. **We want to encourage our children to feel safe telling us anything. If they have to worry about shaping what they say to make it fit with what they think is acceptable to us, there is no safety and no trust.**

If you ask for the truth when you don't know what happened, you must decide whether to believe your child or not by wholly subjective means. It is easy to be mistaken in these circumstances, and your uncertainty will skew the lessons your child might learn. If your child expects that you have already made up your mind about her culpability, then she will understand that what she has to say will have little effect on the verdict, and she will feel that the question is a sham. She learns to disconnect truth from trust, a dangerous lesson, and what is more, she will lose her respect for you.

When we do know what happened in a given situation, we still often ask our children to admit their part. For the child, this feels like a test that cannot be passed. She will feel that no matter what she says, she is a failure, and she will resent you for setting her up in this way. When you ask for – even when you demand – only truth, you are still giving her a choice: to tell the truth or only part of it, or to lie.

You may consider the test a good teaching tool, feeling that when she is rewarded for telling the truth or punished for lying, she will learn the consequences that come with either choice, and will make a better choice the next time. But the child feels betrayed. She feels that, in some sense, you are tempting her with the wrong choice. 'How could you let me do that?' she wonders. Sure, it is her choice, her failure, but you set her up for it. You may know a little more about her from giving the test, but you will have sacrificed a good measure of trust to gain that knowledge.

The other danger in testing a child's truthfulness is that we ourselves may be wrong. We can know the truth without a shadow of a doubt and still be wrong. A funny coincidence proved this to me.

My husband and I were once visiting with friends, who told us that they had found glitter-gold nail polish spilled and dried on the windowsill in their daughter's bedroom. She had denied spilling it. Our friends had pressed her again and again to tell the truth, and when she continued to deny the spill, they lectured her sternly about lying and gave full voice to their displeasure and disappointment.

When we saw them, they were dismayed to think that she would lie to them about something so obvious. They knew she was guilty. Except... she wasn't. As it turned out, we had rented that house before our friends moved into it, and *our* daughter had a bottle of the very same nail polish. She had spilled it, and we were unable to remove it and left it there when we moved out. Their daughter was telling the truth.

Children don't always learn the lessons we intend for them. An expectation that we assume is simple and crystal-clear can seem fraught with contradictions to your child. And trust, which is built slowly over a long time, is easily shattered by one or two mistakes.

Think of it: when someone lies to you, how long does it take afterwards until you can hear that person without a little reservoir of doubt? Do you want to feel that doubt about your child? It is very uncomfortable. And if your child feels unsure about what to say or about how it will be received, she may well be wary of saying anything, let alone the truth. Do you want to risk that?

Using Ho Hum to Foster Honesty and Trust

There is an alternate route, a less risky one that builds trust, encourages honesty, and guides children toward taking responsibility for their own words and actions. The principles of Ho Hum serve as a guide. First: when something happens, consider *not* asking your child to tell you the truth. I don't mean asking her to tell you lies instead, I mean don't ask anything: don't ask about what happened, don't ask about what she did or didn't do, don't ask who else was involved, and don't ask how she could be so stupid, so thoughtless or so intent on turning your hair grey.

Consider *not* telling her how disappointed, embarrassed, angry and upset you are, not telling her how difficult her life will be now that she has shown herself to be untrustworthy, and not telling her about all the limited and nasty employment options she will have available to her if she continues on this path of moral corruption. As potentially serious and true as these predictions are, now is not the time. And yes, it takes a huge – no – it takes a super-human amount of Ho Hum to restrain yourself from saying them.

What *do* you do, if you are not saying those things? You act. You respond to what happened. And this is where you will need as firm a grasp as possible on your reserves of Ho Hum.

Here's an example: Shortly after we moved to New Hampshire, my then fourteen-year-old son, Thomas, made it onto the local high school varsity hockey team. The team was great. The juniors and seniors took him under their wings, giving him a nickname ('Montana') and lots of genuinely useful advice about the game, about working with the enthusiastic and high-intensity coach, and, I am sure, about girls. My son was thrilled to be on this team, to be playing at this level, to be on the ice instead of warming the bench.

High school hockey can be rough, so before the season started we had our son take an Impact test. This establishes a baseline for an athlete's normal level of balance, vision and memory. In the event that a potential concussion occurs, the athlete can retake the test, and the results are compared to his own 'normal' baseline. Concussions are serious injuries that are hard to diagnose, and athletes and their coaches are notorious for trying to downplay the severity of an injury in order to get the athlete back to playing as soon as possible. The Impact test is an objective way to tell whether the athlete has a concussion and when it is safe to return to play.

Two weeks after Thomas took the test, he was elbowed in the head during a game and was flattened. He didn't lose consciousness, but it took him a full minute to get up. The next day he was tired and had a headache. This was not unexpected the day after an intense game, but we decided to have him Impact tested to assess any injury to the brain. His test came back indicating some memory deficits, so he sat out some practices and the next game. While the coach did not insist that Thomas return right away, he did indicate displeasure at losing him for a game.

The biggest danger to the brain is having a second injury before fully recovering from the first one, so athletes should wait for a clear Impact test before returning to the ice. Before the next game, Thomas took the test again. His score indicated a full recovery, so he was cleared to play.

When we got home, I called the coach to let him know that Thomas had been given a green light, and then Thomas and I sat down to work on a Spanish lesson. While we were sitting, Thomas must have had an itch because he lifted up his shirt to rub his stomach, and, lo and behold, what did I see? Two three-letter sequences written upside down on his stomach. 'You cheated!' I blurted out, before being rendered speechless by the implications of what he had done (and being speechless is not a condition I generally suffer from).

As I sat there wrestling with incredulity, Thomas seemed at first to have been taken by surprise, but after a few moments, he gathered himself together and was clearly about to launch into a defense. 'Don't even try,' I growled. 'Out. Take the dog for a walk.' I knew that as soon as he opened his mouth with some lame excuse or far-fetched explanation for what was written on his stomach, I would lose whatever small grasp I had on my Ho Hum, and it would become a festival of angry shouting as I gave vent to my frustration and disappointment about his cheating, as well as my feelings of fear at what might have happened had we let him back on the ice.

With Thomas safely out of range for the moment, I called my husband and fumed. After some colorful moments, we both took a big breath. OK, now what do we do? It was fairly self-evident. He would not be allowed to play until he had been re-tested, at his own expense, and the test had shown he was clear from any effects of the original impact.

After Thomas got back with the dog, he tentatively stuck his head in the door. I looked at him and shrugged in a matter-of-fact 'Now you are really going to have to dig yourself out of this one' sort of way, and he nodded. Then his face fell and tears came, along with an admission. He didn't try to excuse what he had done but instead said that he realized how stupid and dangerous it was. He asked what he needed to do now, I explained, and he agreed that it was what made the most sense. He even seemed relieved that he wouldn't be allowed to play. He knew the risk.

I didn't ask him what had happened, but as we drove up to the rink to explain to the coach and the team why he wouldn't be playing, he told me how pressured he felt, while at the same time acknowledging that the ultimate choice had been his. The more he talked, the more he understood how he had come to make such a bad decision. What a brilliant idea it had seemed to him at the time! A pen in his pocket, he would be alone to take the test. What could possibly go wrong?

I assumed that he had been given some encouragement in this endeavor, but I didn't ask about that either. I did ask him what he thought he could do next time he felt pressured to do something questionable, and I assured him that there would be a next time. He looked a bit daunted by the prospect, given his recent failure, but he came up with a few good ideas, which included talking to us or, if that proved to be too difficult or embarrassing, to his big sister, who is 'cool' but also fiercely protective. That sounded like a good start to me.

When we walked into the rink, none of the normally cheerful and friendly seniors would meet my eye. I don't know for sure, but I am guessing that they told Thomas to do whatever he needed to do to pass the test. It was a huge compliment to him. They wanted him there. Nothing could be more tempting to a fourteen-year-old boy. But it was still his choice and his responsibility, and if he didn't see it then, he certainly did now.

By handling his cheating this way, did I inoculate Thomas from further errors of bad judgment? No. Am I certain that he will not lie in the future? No. While I don't think he will cheat on another Impact test if he needs one, I expect that he will continue to make some mistakes. My Ho Hum response *did* do two things, however: it enabled him to freely recognize and own his responsibility for making a bad choice, and it added another layer to our foundation of trust. Because I avoided (just barely!) an emotional reaction, and didn't give a long lecture, there was nowhere else to put his attention but where it belonged: on the problem he had created. Because we by-passed the interrogation, there was nowhere else to put his energy but into a solution.

Parents can be tempted to punish a child for lying, thinking that if the punishment is sufficiently severe, the child will want to avoid a repeat and will no longer lie. This, unfortunately, is exactly backward. A child who is punished is full of fear, humiliation and anger. The anger diverts the child from considering her own responsibility because she is so focused on the behavior of the parent. The fear prevents her from ever feeling safe enough to tell the parent anything. The child's primary motivation will be to protect herself from the parent she doesn't trust, and in order to do that, she will lie.

When I talk about developing the foundation of trust, I am talking about your child's trust in you, not your trust in your child. Trusting our children is definitely a worthy goal, but we do more harm than good when we put the cart before the horse, expecting honesty before they are sure that *they* can trust *us*. It is possible to skip the part where you ask your child to confess and to keep your focus on the original infraction, the one about which your child might potentially lie. It is our response to *that* event which is so key to developing trust.

Don't give your child the opportunity to lie: don't ask. Resist the temptation to test your child's honesty. It is a work in progress, a tender shoot that needs steady nourishment and gentle care. A stiff wind will just snap it before it has developed the inner strength and the resources to withstand the full force of the elements. Ultimately, your child will be able to withstand great challenges. Use the time you have to build trust. Honesty is a gift your child will eventually bring to you freely, if you wait until she is ready.

Address the original infraction by avoiding blame and focusing on solutions. In our case, this meant focusing on Thomas' cheating. He made a bad choice, and it caused some real problems that required action. Kids make mistakes. They make bad choices. Don't you? With your guidance, you can hope that the mistakes will not be too damaging to your children or others, but even if you were a perfect parent, your child would make mistakes. It is simply part of learning to live.

So if we assume that mistakes will happen, we can respond – Ho Hum – in a way that teaches our children how to remedy the problem that they have created. By doing this instead of testing, blaming or punishing them, we teach our children that we can be relied upon for help. They can come to us with their mistakes, and we will help them figure out how to fix them. They are not off the hook, but they are also not alone. It is safe to tell us, no matter what they did. They will trust us. And when *they* trust *us*, there is less need to lie.

Solutions Rather than Blame

If we are going to seek solutions without asking our children what they've done, we need to be willing to act without knowing all of the truth. We need to be able to act without certainty. When something has gone wrong, you either know that your kid has erred, or you don't. If you know for sure who has done what, you can and should approach it as you would any error that comes up in your presence. And **if you don't know what happened or who is responsible, you should *still* handle it as if you do know: handle it as if it occurred while you were watching. Whoever is there, and that includes everyone, cleans up the mess.**

If you were at the dinner table together and your child spilled milk onto the floor, would you ask her to admit that she had done it – to tell the truth – or would you expect her to clean it up according to her age and ability? I think most of us would bypass the truth test, since we were right there when it happened, and go straight to clean up. (Many of us might add a helping of admonishment to that as well: tempting but counter-productive.)

So when we have not personally witnessed the infraction, why do we ask our kids to tell us the truth about what happened? How will we know what is the truth and what is a lie? As our friends with the glitter nail polish found out, even when we know for sure, we can be wrong. So why do we need to know for sure before we act? Is it because we want to pin the blame on someone? Is it because we don't want the guilty party to get away with something? Is it because we want to feel reassured that we are acting justly?

If we respond to the misdeed as a mistake – a mistaken act, a mistaken way of thinking – then we have no need to punish, so the worry that the wrong person might be punished or the guilty person escape punishment is no longer relevant. A mistake calls for some sort of action to fix it, guidance about how to handle the situation in the future, and possibly a consequence. A problem has arisen, and we all gather our forces to right it.

But what if we are wrong in assigning responsibility, as our friends were in the case of the spilled nail polish? Well, let's consider what might have happened if they had handled the spill as a mistake, instead of asking for the 'truth' and then blaming their daughter not only for the spill but for lying about it as well. Let's say that they found the spill and went to their daughter, described the problem, collected cleaning supplies and together cleaned it up. They might also have decided that they needed to put the nail polish away and their daughter would only be able to use it with supervision. Ho Hum. No blame. This is just the way it is right now.

The daughter might respond in several ways. She might say, 'That is not my nail polish on the sill. I didn't spill it, so why do I have to clean it up?' The issue is not about who spilled it, but is more about taking care of it. The nail polish is in her room. It makes sense that she clean it up. We need to be responsible for our own space. Rather than teaching our kids to police others' behavior, we should teach them to focus on their own.

If the parents don't put undue focus on the daughter's guilt, she will not put undue focus on protecting herself from the accusation. She won't have to lie to evade their punishment and disappointment, since the focus is on action, on the solution.

If she did spill the polish, well, all the more reason to clean it up. If she didn't, she can still feel good about cleaning it up since it repairs something in her own room. If children feel good about taking part in the solution, they are much more willing to continue to contribute to the collective sorting out of problems in the future – whether they are the cause or not. There is no blame. Blaming is a distraction from the real issue at hand: how are we going to take care of this? If parents respond with Ho Hum instead of with angry and judgmental blaming, everyone's energy can be directed toward the solution, not toward the person who made the mistake.

Sometimes, in an effort to encourage their kids to admit the truth, parents will offer a trade: if the child tells the truth, she will be treated lightly. This is a mistake. The child may, in some sense, be relieved that she will not be taken to task for her error, but in her heart, she knows that this bargain is a bit shady. Admission of guilt does not necessarily lead to contrition. It is the remedial action taken to fix the problem caused by her error or the amends made on behalf of the people that she has hurt which brings absolution.

It is said that the truth shall set one free. Yes, it will, if the truth is offered willingly, but not if it is admitted grudgingly out of fear or in order to take advantage of a free pass. If we teach our children and teens to squarely face their mistakes and bad choices, to discern what needs to be done to make things right, and to throw themselves into this meaningful work, then we will have given them a clear path towards redemption. Being trustworthy doesn't mean being perfect. It means being responsible for one's mistakes as well as one's successes. **When we have shown our children that we can be trusted, they will bring us the truth unasked, at first to get our help, and later, to show us that they don't need help anymore.**

Asking for the truth has different implications at different ages:

Under Seven

A child under seven years old wants to believe that you know everything. When you ask her to tell the truth, you are indicating that you don't know. This is unsettling to her, as she feels most secure when she assumes that you know all and will handle it, including her transgressions, with wisdom and aplomb. This is an essential lesson for which your child will ever be grateful: any crisis can be handled. There is a solution, and you, the parent, will help her find it.

Ages Seven to Fourteen

At this stage the reins are loosening just a bit. Your child's opportunities and experience will broaden, and there is much more room for error. There will be mistakes. This is the time when your consistency is crucial. Just as you would with any other choice at this stage, avoid offering the unacceptable option of lying by skipping the truth test and going right to action – response.

As your child becomes aware that you are not, in fact, all-powerful, she will be keenly aware of her own imperfections as well. Will you still see the beauty and goodness in her, despite her moments of bad judgment and worse behavior? Has the world changed irrevocably when she makes a mistake? Can she still rely on you to help her sort out her scrapes?

Keeping your grasp of Ho Hum and focusing on remedies and reasonable consequences instead of blame and punishment will encourage her to develop her sense of personal responsibility instead of developing her techniques for self-defense. You will be rewarded for your efforts: your child will enter the tumultuous time of adolescence bonded to you with love, respect and – most elusive – trust.

Ages Fourteen and Over

As teenagers move out into the world, they forge powerful relationships with other people. It is a considerable challenge for them to balance their commitments to school, family and friends. They must learn to juggle their sometimes competing loyalties as well as all the demands on their time. In addition, they feel driven to seek the absolute truth in all things, but while they are compelled to see all things in black and white, the world does not cooperate. Instead, it shows itself as mostly grey; there are multiple truths.

As they struggle to navigate through these contradictions, we parents can offer an unyielding reef of judgment and blame against which they will throw all their resistance, or we can offer a guiding beacon of light. They must ultimately find their own way, but the light can help. It reminds them that they are capable, that they don't need to panic, that they can do what they have always done when the going gets rough, even if the storm seems more overwhelming than they ever imagined or prepared for. Knowing that you are there and that you see them struggling is not something to fear and hide from but is a relief, a refuge. They know, they trust, that when they arrive on shore, no matter how battered and wrecked they are, you will be there, still shining for them.

Chapter Twelve
Sibling Conflict

Squabbling among siblings is a huge source of headaches for parents. It is aggravating and distressing when our children fight. We want them to get along and to love each other and for their relationship to be supportive and flexible enough to last a lifetime. It is hard to imagine that happening when they are at each other's throats, in a rage, flinging fists or insults at each other's weak spots in the way only a brother or sister knows how to do. We want it to stop, and so we think that if we go to the heart of it – the source of the conflict – and get that settled, then all will be well again. Peace and harmony will be restored. Without the conflict, we think, there will no longer be any need for fighting. If only that were true, but of course, it is much more complicated than that.

Conflict is not the problem. **Conflict, on its barest face, is never the problem: conflict is simply the challenge of finding a way for more than one need or want or perspective to exist. In a word, it is about being different, and there is nothing inherently wrong with that.** Can you imagine how dull the world would be if we were all exactly alike in every way? Can you imagine being married to yourself, having yourself over for a visit, raising yourself? Hopefully you like yourself enough that this prospect isn't a total horror, but really, the conversations would start to feel a little tedious. It is precisely the conflict that arises from our difference from each other that makes life interesting, that propels us forward and that challenges us to learn and grow. If we are uncomfortable with conflict or if we don't know how to deal with it, then that can lead to arguments and worse.

Conflict among siblings is inevitable, and arguments follow for many reasons, chief among them being children's lack of skills in resolving conflict in a positive way. They often have a deep and broad skill-set for resolving it in a negative way, and I don't think I need to list any of those for you here. **Unwittingly, and with all good intentions, parents often respond to conflict in ways that not only encourage their children to continue to fight, but fail, in the actions and experiences they give their children, to teach crucial lessons about handling conflict.**

Where do they go wrong? Some avoid the whole issue of guidance and just try to put a stop to the fighting. They escalate the drama by yelling and punishing. Others try to take a more positive approach. They divide up the last cupcake into equal pieces or come up with some sort of solution that they deem to be fair, thinking that this provides a good model of a positive outcome. Or they try to encourage their children, right then and there, to be gentle, to use their words instead of their fists, and so on. These parents are attempting to model a good process.

The parent who punishes children for fighting causes more problems than she solves. All of the usual trouble associated with punishment will be present, and the children receive no guidance about how to resolve their conflict. The more positive approaches have significant merit, but when the chips are down, when the argument is heated or prolonged or is the same one that the children have every day, then a slightly different approach will help.

We need to sweat the small stuff, maintaining the basic boundaries of safety, responsibility and respect, while letting our children wrestle with finding solutions. The motivations and issues, the details and permutations involved in sibling fighting are complicated and endless. Mercifully, what we as parents can do to respond to the infinite variety of arguments and scuffles is relatively simple. Once you have found your Ho Hum – calm parental authority – acting involves two basic elements:

1. Provide physical and emotional space for your children to cool off.
2. Treat your children as a unit.

Provide Physical and Emotional Space

A girl and her little brother are sitting at opposite ends of the sofa. She is reading a book, and he is zooming his little toy car up and around the arm, over the back and around the edge of the bottom cushion. On one of the car's passes, it skids off course and bumps into her foot. 'Sto-op,' she says, without looking up from her book. With louder engine noises this time, he zooms the car right up her shin. She slams down her book, glares at him and shouts, 'I told you to stop. If you touch me again, I'm going to take your car and flush it down the toilet!' Her brother, half-smiling and half-frowning, grabs her book and throws it on the floor, and with a shout of outrage, she reaches for his car and yanks it out of his hand. Wailing in anger and distress, he grabs a pillow and swings it at her, catching her eye in the process. Tears of pain and outrage fill her eyes, as she cries out, 'Mo-om. He hit me.'

Now, the mom who is solution-oriented might come in and divide up the real estate, admonishing them both to stay on their own sides of the sofa and keep their hands to themselves, and explain, very reasonably, that there is plenty of room for each. That's fair. But it is unlikely to solve the problem, since they both are so mad at each other that they will likely continue to needle each other, leading to another blow-up.

The process-oriented mom might come in and tell the brother, 'We don't hit. Use your words,' while saying to the sister, 'Let him know how you feel.' Perhaps she expects her to be able to say something like, 'When you hit me, I feel very upset.' The mother might even make a suggestion, modeling for her child what she could say and how to say it – in a calm, sweet voice. The problem is: that is *not* how the girl feels. She is *mad*, she wants *revenge* and she wants her little brother to *suffer*. Her mother's calm words do not even remotely do justice to how she feels. The little brother, in the meanwhile, is equally upset, and if he were to express himself with words his sister really might not like what she heard.

The original conflict is no longer the issue. Emotions are boiling, and a reasonable solution is out of reach – not because one doesn't exist, but because at this point neither party is interested in a reasonable

178

solution. What the situation calls for now is not a settlement of the conflict, but a settling of emotions. Just like adults, when children are very upset, they will act unreasonably. What reason they have is unavailable to them when they are awash in a sea of emotion.

What they need is Ho Hum. And you can help them make the first rudimentary steps toward Ho Hum in an active, concrete and physical way by giving them time and space to cool off: create some physical space between the situation and their emotions.

Provide time, space and comfort. They will learn that the business of settling the conflict has not been abandoned but is only waiting until they are in a better place to address it – when they are not so hot with anger or blind with hurt. Help them through this process.

It is really tempting to try to 'talk them down.' Resist this temptation. Comfort with hugs, with warmth, with physical gestures, but if you must use words, make them nonsense words, 'There, there.' Especially as your children get older, you will be tempted to jump the gun, to start talking before they have become settled enough, and you will find yourself quickly sucked into the argument, perhaps even becoming a new target. Your action is called for; save your words. **If you can separate your children and give them enough emotional space to cool down, this alone is often enough.**

In the case of the sofa, you could set both children in separate chairs, or if that is not far enough away from each other, in separate rooms, which maintains safety: they can't hurt each other if they can't get to each other. This removal also contracts their freedom: they cannot return to the sofa until they can show that they can do so respectfully.

You have remained calm, and you have acted by giving them space. They are arriving at some level of calmness, and then it is time for them to act, which means finding a solution that works for both. Truthfully, once enough time has passed for emotions to settle, the original conflict has often faded from memory, and when you suggest that you all sit down to figure out a solution, your children, having moved on, will look at you quizzically and say, 'Huh?'

But in the event that the conflict is still there, a solution must be found. When you feel that they are ready, you can gather them together to work out a way forward. When my children were still quite young, I thought that the first step toward a solution was listening: not to me, but to each other. I thought that they could try to express themselves in a non-confrontational way. I learned that this sort of communication took much more time and modeling before they were ready to attempt it themselves. Meanwhile it risks a return to the wrongs and the blaming and the anger. What worked better in the earlier years was to acknowledge, quite matter-of-factly, that there had been a problem and that they had both been very upset and angry. **Name the basic issue of conflict, name the emotions, and then move forward. No blame, no judgment, just statements of fact.** And another statement of fact: 'Before you both can go back to the sofa, you will need to find a solution...' And another statement of fact, '... that you both can agree to.' And one last: 'I am confident that you can figure it out.' And with that, withdraw as much as possible. Let them hash it out.

It will be tempting to suggest possible solutions and to arbitrate between them. Resist! They need you to stay out, to stay neutral and be above it, otherwise they will try to angle for your support and you will become a new source of conflict. **Limit yourself to stating the boundaries. You can veto anything that is egregiously unsafe, irresponsible or disrespectful, but try to be open to what they come up with, if they are both in agreement.** Their own solutions, although they may seem unorthodox, petty or just plain ineffective, have the magic and enhancing ingredient of ownership.

And if it all falls apart, and the argument is rejoined, that does not mean failure at all. It just means that they need still more space before attempting to arrive at a solution. That is not a cause for shame or disappointment. It is simply reality. So provide them the space that they still obviously need. They can try again later. That is, realistically, all you can do. You – and they – cannot force it. No blame, no judgment, no comment. Ho Hum.

Sometimes children – well, let's admit it: all of us – bicker or otherwise behave poorly because we are feeling tired or bored or hungry or just irritable and stressed. It can be important to recognize the reasons, to understand what has driven us or them to fussing or arguing so that we can try to do what we can to address the source of the discomfort by having a snack, going to bed earlier, and so on. But those reasons should never be used as an excuse. We are always responsible for our actions, no matter what the reasons behind them.

Obviously, we want to try to avoid putting our children in this sort of spot by making sure they eat and sleep well, by not overloading them with activities and so on. But **even when we do our best, there will be times when life is just difficult. Recognize those moments, and remind yourself and your children that it is precisely these times when it is hardest to be kind to each other, to be patient and to be respectful, but that it is precisely these times for which manners were invented.** Remind them, gently, that these are the times that call for extra effort. Pool your resources of strength and good humor, and share them back out, like crumbs at the bottom of the barrel on a long voyage. Keep your eyes on the horizon and peeled for land, 'Only ten more minutes and we'll be home!' **Be intrepid together and hold back the forces of grumpiness.**

Treat Your Children as a Unit

Let's return to our sofa scenario. The mom has walked in just as the little brother swings the pillow at his sister's head. He is obviously guilty. She has seen it with her own eyes. But what has she missed? When she turns her focus on him, he will cry out, 'But she took my car!' And the sister, older and more sophisticated, will say, dismissively, 'Well, he started it. I was just sitting there reading my book.'

She is feeling smug and vindicated. He is the likely suspect, and Mom is an eyewitness to his crime. But what Mom didn't see was that before any of the incidents with the car, the little brother asked his sister what she was reading and she sneered at him, saying, 'Nothing that stupid little brothers need to know.' Now, of course, they are both responsible for their own behavior, no matter how sorely they are provoked. It is not that the little brother isn't guilty. It is that the sister is guilty, too.

We parents will never know the whole story. What we see may indeed be only the final chapter of a long and convoluted story. When we respond to sibling conflict, we want to be fair, but how can we when we don't have all the information? We can't. By assigning blame or responsibility to one sibling, there is an even chance that we will be

181

wrong. By treating them all as a unit, there is as good a chance that a relatively 'innocent' child will be roped into working out a solution and possibly even having her boundaries contracted along with those of the more 'guilty' sibling. Yes, you, the parent, might err in that. But if you do not treat them all the same by contracting the boundaries of all of them, there is a good chance that you will contract the boundary of the wrong one.

Put yourself in your children's shoes: which would be worse? In their eyes, blind justice (treating them all alike, even if it means treating them all equally wrong) is far better than injustice (picking the wrong one). If you try to pick, you will be wrong some of the time. Your children will not go easy on you for this. They will not see it as your genuine efforts to be fair and just. They will interpret it as favoritism, and there is nothing worse than that for sibling relationships.

When I was young, maybe six or so, I got into a fight with my little sister over poker chips (my grandfather's: we loved to stack the different colors and make patterns). It ended up with her biting me and me hitting her back. My mother, hearing the ruckus, came into the room just as I walloped my sister. I was hauled off to do time, and my little sister was comforted, despite the fact (which I, of course, loudly tried to draw attention to) that there was a giant and livid bite mark on my arm. It was not that I was wrongly accused. It was that she got off scot-free. My resentment was short-lived, but the thing is, I still remember it, not because of the argument, but because of the feeling of injustice. It obviously made an impression.

We need to avoid blaming and to focus instead on identifying the problem, finding a solution and moving forward. **When siblings fight, we need to treat them all as a single unit, regardless of who did what or who 'started' it.** Since the conflict involves both, the solution will necessarily involve both. Frankly, assigning blame is a waste of time and distracts from the task at hand. Your children benefit from unity, from being expected to sink or swim together. One sibling is not singled out as more special than another, and neither is any one sibling manoeuvred to the sidelines. We shift the focus from blame to finding solutions.

In Montana, I had a response to sibling fighting that embodied the two basic principles (give them space; treat them as a unit) in a slightly unorthodox way. Once my children were old enough, I would send them out to walk the pasture fence when they fought with each other. It took about twenty minutes to make the trip around, and in that time I would have my own emotions under control, which is the real first step back to harmony. I sent them out together, and at the start I could see them stomping along, fuming, one often walking way ahead of the other.

But as they came back around, I could tell from the movement of their bodies that they were feeling more relaxed. Their arms swung freely, their stride lengthened, they looked up and around at things. And they were laughing. They would come in the door at the same time, making a commotion with stomping snow off their boots and throwing mittens and hats onto the dryer, their lilting voices talking over and around one another like a stream running over rocks. The original conflict? They had moved forward from it, and together, with pink cheeks and shining eyes, they would head for the refrigerator for a snack to fill the hole in their bellies that the fresh air and exercise had opened up. In the event that they were mad at me, they were unified. I was willing to live with that.

There are an infinite number of issues, snags and conflicts that any given family will have to face. You will have to make adjustments to the general principles outlined here in order to fit you, your children, your priorities and your values. Just remember that conflict is not a cause for despair. It is an opportunity to learn important things about each other, as individuals and as parts of a whole. It is an opportunity for your children to practice handling these challenges with your help, before they go out on their own.

Chapter Thirteen
Every Tendency has a Positive Aspect

Part Three has been about our children misbehaving, challenging boundaries, fighting and having tantrums. While it is important to have a plan for responding to misbehavior, we can do more than simply manage it. We can also try to understand what our children are telling us when they misbehave, and one way to do this is to search for and consider the positive side of difficult behavior. We need to be cautious about leaping from what our children do to who they are, but their behavior will give us, only too clearly sometimes, a sense of their common tendencies. Be confident that any tendency will have light aspects as well as dark ones, constructive possibilities as well as destructive ones. Difficult behavior, mistakes and frustrations give us the opportunity to see and understand the whole of our children more clearly and to find better ways to channel their behavior in a positive direction.

When my son Thomas was about eighteen months old, he loved to whack things. My mother would call and ask, 'How is O'Thomas doing today?' because whenever I was on the phone with her (in other words, distracted), my son would inevitably end up whacking something, and I would say, 'Oh, Thomas' as I headed over to pick things up, redirect him and take away the spatula or whatever.

The nickname was an acknowledgment that he was a bit troublesome, but the humor in it, as is so often the case, helped me to defer judgment and respond to the immediate issue of the moment without feeling the crushing pressure to 'fix' him.

As well as whacking things, he liked to toss my mixing bowls over the side of our second-story deck to see what happened when they landed. Luckily, the bowls were metal and were usable even while dented, but it is a considerable pain to have to hike around the house in search of your cooking utensils every time you want to mix up a batch of pancakes.

Was his behavior bad? Was he bad himself? Frankly, 'bad' didn't have anything to do with it. It *never* does. Was his behavior an immediate problem? Yes. Every object in the house was at risk of being either whacked or used to whack something else. Was the behavior destructive? Yes. Did I have to attend to his behavior? Yes.

If I had judged his behavior as bad, I might have been tempted to respond harshly in an attempt to eradicate it. If I decided that since he was good at heart his behavior must therefore be good as well, I might have been tempted to let it go – to tell myself that he was just 'expressing' himself. When I suspended judgment, when I could just observe the situation with curiosity – Ho Hum – I saw that Thomas was simply a little boy with a lot of physical energy, and while he might well have been expressing himself with that energy, he was causing damage in the process. Was I going to limit that self-expression? You bet. He could express himself all he wanted: outside, where it would cause no harm. Inside, there were limits to what he could bang and what he could use to bang with. No judgment. No comment, either. If he started whacking the toilet seat with a wooden spoon, the spoon was taken away or switched with something softer. And we spent a lot of time outside. (People used to wonder why my vegetable garden was so large – now you know.) There, he could whack things to his heart's content.

Depending on the context, Thomas's tendency to burn off a lot of physical energy could be good or bad, useful or a nuisance. On the surface, all that whacking was pretty destructive. If I couldn't have looked beyond what was immediately apparent to the eye, I would have assumed that my boy was destructive, in other words bad. But by suspending judgment, by taking the time to consider, I could see the tendency behind the behavior and redirect it towards constructive activity.

By the time he was three, Thomas was using that physical energy to help move dirt with his boy-sized wheelbarrow. He shoveled snow like a champion, forked manure out of the barn with gusto, and dug fencepost holes with focus and determination. Did he still leave a swath of destruction behind him? Rarely.

185

As parents we can dig beneath misbehavior to find the tendency beneath. We can draw out that supposed weakness to the light and find a context in which it becomes a strength. Remember, your child has been born with everything she needs. She just has to learn how best to work with it. She must recognize the value of the qualities and tendencies that make her herself, and understand how they can help or hinder her. This is a lifelong challenge, and she will need you to lead the way.

With time, attention and patience we may be able to channel that tendency in a way that ennobles it: elevates it, welcomes it and treats it with dignity. Since neither you nor anyone else can change the fundamental being of your child, it is your challenge is help her learn how to use what she has in a positive way. You must help her to know herself, to develop all that she has, to be more herself instead of trying to shut parts away. It can take a long time for the good in a tendency to be realized. More than anything, your child needs you to have faith in her and in her potential.

Here's an example of what I mean by seeing and ennobling a tendency. My daughter sets extraordinarily high standards for herself and because she works so hard, she accomplishes great things. She took up ballet when she was younger, and reached a surprisingly high level despite coming from a small, rural town with a delightfully modest and decidedly recreational dance school.

Ballet is demanding, and she embraced the discipline and the life wholeheartedly, her leg extended out with her foot up on the bathroom counter as she brushed her teeth, her back and neck tall and straight and graceful as she sat at the table eating while the rest of us slouched and shoveled in food.

'Work hard *and* have fun,' was our motto. But in her drive for mastery, she became more aware of the ideal and even more keenly aware of the gap between herself and that ideal. At times it appeared that she could no longer see what she had, but could only see the tiny bit she didn't have.

I had tried to focus on the positive, to reinforce what she had accomplished, how talented she was, how she had persevered through considerable difficulty and challenge. But I realized, one day, after she had come to me and was sitting on my bed, her lovely cheek bent in utter sorrow and defeat, that I had missed the whole point. I, with all my love and my good intentions, had been trying to emphasize what I saw as the positive in her. But what I had not done, what she needed me to do, was to ennoble that which was negative. She needed me to drag, albeit gently, but drag nevertheless, that which was a darkness in her out into the light and find a way to make it good.

Nina's keen perception, her ability to understand where the weaknesses are, her willingness to see the whole truth, not just the pleasant truth, could be of great value, but the problem came from her directing that knowing eye solely on herself. Like a mirror concentrating the sun's rays, she had been the focus of all that attention, and just as if it were the sun, it was scorching her. But what if she were to turn that focus elsewhere? What if, instead of denying that part of herself, she was to use it? Harness it? What if she became *more* herself, instead of trying to become less?

The opportunity came in the form of the yearly recital that the local dance school organized each spring. Nina's dance teacher asked if she would be interested in helping to choreograph and teach a dance to a class of young girls. The music was a waltz from *Swan Lake*. The class, while having several years of ballet under their belts, were still very much beginners, but oh, did those girls want to be ballerinas.

Nina accepted the invitation (thank you, Miss Elizabeth), and we watched as this group of gangling girls transformed themselves into swans, but even better, we watched as our daughter filled with a radiant glow. She explained to me later what she had been doing. She went into the class and while she and the dance teacher worked out steps, Nina observed the girls. She watched them while they stood at the barre. She watched them while they waited in line to skip and leap across the floor. She watched them before class as they were putting up their hair and gossiping. She knew who was chatty, who was strong, who really felt the music, and who was there in body but not mind. And she ennobled them all.

She designed a part for each girl that would spotlight her particular strength, and, most of all, she inspired them with her own grace and carriage. I will tell you, when those girls appeared on stage, they did not stride to their places and open their arms in preparation, as the other classes did. They glided onstage, opened their wings, settled their feathers, and when the music began, they were alive, they were beautiful and serene, and they knew it. Perfect technique? Not even close. Perfect performance? The best I have seen.

My daughter is learning to bring her ability to see what is missing and what is needed to those who benefit from such intense attention. It seems that when she is challenged to meet the needs of others, her perfectionism evaporates and she works to draw out the best from those around her, enabling them to feel beautiful and capable.

She learned to take a tendency that was dark, and rather than fight it or try to remove it, she found a context where it could be light. Our children need us to foster these ennobling opportunities for them and with them. Rather than judging them, we need to truly and patiently see them.

Praise and Self-Esteem

While we are discussing taking the time to really see our children clearly, here's a quick note about praise.

Most children receive a lot of praise. They hear 'good job' so often it has become almost meaningless. When children are praised left and right, they learn that they are constantly under the spotlight. This is particularly problematic for children under age seven, who develop best when they are not pressured to an early consciousness or heightened awareness of self. The feeling that they are constantly being evaluated and judged, that they are constantly on display, can lead to a dependence on approval. The approval, the praise itself, becomes the source of motivation, rather than the child's own sense of pleasure and satisfaction.

Also, praise that focuses on outcomes or on the child's identity ('You're a great speller!') rather than on effort can leave her lost when tasks become more challenging or she is not doing so well.

How can we encourage our children without falling into these traps? Praise is best when the majority of it is disconnected from judgment. That is not a typo. Praise that lifts children, allows them to feel real satisfaction with themselves and encourages them to keep at something relies on **description, not evaluation**. When you describe what you see – a drawing or a turn at bat or a gesture of friendship to a new kid – you are showing your child that you see *her*, that *she* is what matters, not just the results of what she did. Instead of feeling judged, she feels recognized.

Try:

* 'You got so many right!' instead of 'You're a great speller!'
* 'You rode your bike all the way from the corner!' instead of 'Great ride!'
* 'You stuck with it until you got it done' instead of 'Good job!'
* 'Look at all of those colors. I see blues and reds and purples...' instead of 'What a great drawing!'
* 'That other player really wanted to provoke you, but you kept your cool. You really care about sportsmanship' instead of 'Good game.'
* 'You remembered to bring your jacket home,' instead of 'Good girl.'
* 'Thank you' instead of 'You are such a good helper.'
* 'I laughed when I read your story' instead of 'Great story!'

With Ho Hum we can respond to the challenges children inevitably bring to us. We can treat their misbehavior as mistakes from which they can learn and through which we will guide them. We can be calm and authoritative, and we can act to give them experiences that help them make changes in their behavior: that allow them to make amends, to reflect, to feel the connection between freedom and responsibility, to recover from tantrums, to come to us honestly with their problems, to negotiate conflict.

We can also observe our children and their tendencies with warmth and curiosity so that over time we can understand the positive aspect of tendencies that are causing problems. We can find ways to channel their behavior in that positive direction. Our children need us to be relentless in this quest to find their unrealized potential for good. When we ennoble what is troublesome or challenging in our children, we show them that we are willing to know them and embrace them in their wholeness. That willingness is a great parental gift: it shines a powerful guiding light on each child's own path toward self-discovery.

Conclusion

Chapter Fourteen
Ho Hum in *Your* Family Life

Is the mother always to blame? When children are behaving in challenging ways, is it because of their parenting? It can be very hard to hear that some of the choices that we make as parents may be contributing to a difficulty. Yet there's no way of being a parent without confronting this possibility at times. Here is the thing: when Copernicus studied the heavens and determined that the Earth did in fact orbit around the sun, he overlooked one important fact of life – mothers are the center of the universe. You know it. You can't blink, you can't take a nap, you can't give a hug or make an idle comment without it rippling out to all those around you. What you do matters: always, and to everyone. It is the relentlessness of that responsibility that makes mothering, parenting, caring for children so exhausting and so challenging.

The considerable weight of that responsibility can feel like a burden some days. Sometimes we are just flattened. But the beauty of it – our salvation – is that because mothers are at the center of it all, we can make adjustments, even small adjustments, and they too will ripple out to those around us. Our smallest shifts can have profound effects: not shifts in who we are, but adjustments in what we do and say. Does that mean we have control over everything and are responsible for every aspect of who our children are and what they do? No, thank goodness. It means that we have a big part to play. We matter. Just a little ray of clarity will show that we have what we need within ourselves. We are enough.

OK, so now what? It was my hope in having this conversation with you that we might put aside some of the roadblocks that make raising children harder than it needs to be, or, at the least, that we might identify the big trouble spots so that you are not taken by surprise when you meet them along the way. While I am hoping that you feel empowered, it is also possible that you are feeling overwhelmed. Perhaps you feel that you have already become hopelessly lost. Perhaps you feel regret for taking a different path than the one you might choose now, were you back at that crossroads again.

First of all, I would say with absolute sincerity, 'Welcome to the club.' We are all members. But I would also remind you that it is not your job to be perfect. It is your job to do the best you can with what you have at the moment. If circumstances change or you learn something new, then you can make an adjustment if you can. That is all you can do. You are who you are, and your challenge is to find the best way of working with what you have. You will find that it (your full self) will serve you well, if you let it. That is what striving is, and you must show your children how to do this, how to get up each day and start again, because they are not perfect either, and they too must learn to live in the world given who they are.

And who is to say what the right path is? It may be that the very tangle in which you find yourself holds something crucial for you or your child. The perspective that I have laid out here for you is only useful insofar as it helps you. If it doesn't help, ditch it. Of course I want to be helpful, but more so, I want to recognize *you*. I want to say to you, 'I see you trying.'

What if you *would* like to make some adjustments? Where can you start? The first thing to remember is to focus on making a change in what you *do*, not who you *are*. The second thing to remember is to focus on yourself, not your children and not your spouse. It is so tempting, when we want to make some adjustments, to look around and say, 'Well, things are going to be a bit different from now on, and let's start with *you*.'

Your child will likely do some things differently in response to what you do. That is all fine and good and can be one of the goals. By all means, discuss what you are thinking with your spouse, but do not expect him or her to immediately jump on the bandwagon, and, more importantly, avoid making him or her into the object of your improvement project. The change originates with you. It is all about you and what you do or don't do.

194

Starting Small

Start small. Pick one thing. Even better: pick one small part of one thing. Every tiny adjustment you make will create ripples that grow and expand outward to all of those around you. And there will be a domino effect: making one small shift will set others in motion, and you will find that many things fall into place with very little effort on your part. So take it slowly. Make one tiny adjustment and give it a month or two to percolate. Where do the ripples reach? There really isn't one best place to start; wherever *you* start is the best place. The important thing is to make that one step.

Attributed to Goethe, the following sums up what I mean about all that flows from taking the first step:

> Until one is committed, there is hesitancy, the chance
> to draw back. Concerning all acts of initiative (and
> creation), there is one elementary truth, the ignorance of
> which kills countless ideas and splendid plans: that the
> moment one definitely commits oneself, then Providence
> moves too. All sorts of things occur to help one that
> would never otherwise have occurred. A whole stream
> of events issues from the decision, raising in one's favor
> all manner of unforeseen incidents and meetings and
> material assistance, which no man could have dreamed
> would have come his way. Whatever you can do, or dream
> you can do, begin it. Boldness has genius, power and
> magic in it. Begin it now.

Ten Questions You Can Ask Yourself

Every child, every parent and every family is unique. What I have tried to explain here in this book are general principles, which you will have to tailor to your own specific problems and challenges. To help you do that, the following is a list of questions that you can ask yourself as you search for the path that is right for you.

1. What lack of clarity/understanding/skill (in me, in my child) has led to this?
2. What is my child seeking?
3. What tendency is present here (in me, in my child)? How can that tendency be ennobled?
4. What emotional gesture does my child need?
5. How can I adjust the family rhythm to better support our life as a family?
6. How can I structure the environment to better support our life as a family?
7. How can I act to guide my child? What am I saying, and how can I substitute action for words?
8. What is the boundary, and is it clear to everyone?
9. How can I model the behavior that I want to see, and where am I modeling the behavior I don't want to see?
10. Where is the humor in the situation? The joy? The warmth? The love?

If You Are Still Stuck

Sometimes, asking yourself questions is not enough. There may be times when you are so overwhelmed by fear that no amount of figuring out will do. When all else fails and you are lying awake, tortured with worry, here is something else you can try. Draw an image in your mind of your child – not the child you wish for, but the child you have. Imagine him or her bathed in the light of your love. Don't worry about imagining your child with strength or power or some sort of desired quality. Picture your child surrounded by love, because even if it only comes from you, that is real. Go to sleep, if you do sleep, with this image. Do this for several nights if you can, and you may find that in the morning, there has been some small shift, some small ripple that has allowed you to glimpse a possibility, a trail of crumbs that you can follow, however tentatively at first.

And you might do the same for yourself now and then: imagine yourself bathed in love, full of love for your children – not an image of you, the superhero, fixing it all, but you, just as you are and full of love, because that is after all, the beginning and the end, your strength and your weakness, the seed and the soil.

The End and the Beginning

We begin the journey of raising our children with each child literally a part of our selves. In our bodies and then in our arms, we carry them, snug, curled into our warmth, feeling the beat of our hearts and the strength of our love and protection. Somehow, as we travel along, past the place where our children must hold our hands to balance; past the place where they run ahead a bit and then rush back to us, trembling; past the place where they set off on a side trail to meet us farther along with the light of adventure and triumph in their eyes; somewhere, we come to a place where we realize that we no longer walk the same path.

Our paths will cross. We will still walk together at times, keeping good company. We may find that they still need us, every now and then, to shine some light so that they can find their way. We may find them unexpectedly at our sides, an arm slipping companionably through ours when we falter. But an earthquake of untold magnitude has happened while we were busy attending to each day, and the whole landscape has shifted beneath us. Our hearts leap with joy and a momentary desolation. Our children are no longer ours. They belong to themselves and have their own journeys ahead of them. But they are not lost to us. No, we are only beginning a new journey, where we see each other with the warmth and wonder of genuine recognition, where we courageously offer and gratefully accept the true gift of self.

Calm Kids

Help Children Relax with Mindful Activities

Lorraine E. Murray

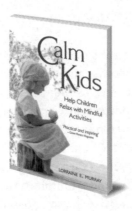

'In this practical and inspiring book, Lorraine Murray shows how to lead fun and peaceful meditation sessions with children.'
– *The Green Parent*

Mindfulness and meditation can help children recognise and cope with modern pressures, giving them simple tools to deal with tension and stress throughout their lives.

Lorraine explains a variety of different approaches, from meditations around daily activities for busy families, to ideas for group 'quietness' sessions in schools. She provides fun, tactile rhymes for toddlers to help them calm down before bedtime, and suggests ways to help teenagers reduce anxiety. She goes on to explain how these methods can help children with ADHD and those on the autistic spectrum, giving a range of case studies.

This book is suitable for complete beginners, or those with some experience of relaxation and meditation techniques. It offers all the advice needed to lead sessions which will help children to feel calmer, happier and more peaceful.

 Also available as an eBook

www.florisbooks.co.uk

Happy Child, Happy Home
Conscious Parenting and Creative Discipline
Lou Harvey-Zahra

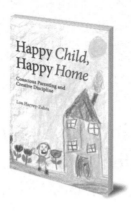

'This is a fantastic parenting book, just for the sheer fact that it aims to encourage happiness and positivity in children and families...
As a mum to two children under the age of three, I found this parenting guide very relevant to my children's stages of development, and the light and friendly tone made for enjoyable reading too.
Families Rating: 6 out of 6 stars.'
– *Families Online, November 2014*

This practical and inspiring book introduces 'conscious parenting' as a new way of helping any family home become more harmonious.

Lou Harvey-Zahra, an experienced parenting coach and teacher, wants to help parents develop calm and happy children. Drawing her inspiration from a Steiner-Waldorf background, she offers candid, relevant and funny tips and advice for taking a clear look at family life, identifying what's not working, and exploring new ideas for improving parent-child relationships.

 Also available as an eBook

www.florisbooks.co.uk

You may also be interested in these parenting titles

Stress-Free Parenting in 12 Steps
Christiane Kutik

Why Children Don't Listen
A Guide for Parents and Teachers
Monika Kiel-Hinrichsen

You and Your Teenager
Understanding the Journey
Jeanne Meijs

A Guide to Child Health
A Holistic Approach to Raising Healthy Children
Dr Michaela Glöckler & Dr Wolfgang Goebel

Vaccination
A Guide for Making Personal Choices
Dr Hans-Peter Studer & Dr Geoffrey Douch

Pregancy, Birth and Beyond
A Spiritual and Practical Guide
Erika Gradenwitz-Koehler